the glimpse of you
was a delight

Pete

glimpse

glimpse

text by Pete Sarsfield

photos by Bob Jeffery

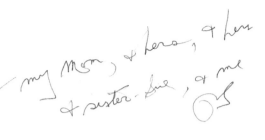

Note for Librarians: A cataloguing record for this book is available from Library and Archives Canada at www.collectionscanada.ca/amicus/index-e.html
ISBN 1-4251-1180-7

Printed in Victoria, BC, Canada. Printed on paper with minimum 30% recycled fibre. Trafford's print shop runs on "green energy" from solar, wind and other environmentally-friendly power sources.

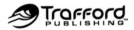

Offices in Canada, USA, Ireland and UK

Book sales for North America and international:
Trafford Publishing, 6E–2333 Government St.,
Victoria, BC V8T 4P4 CANADA
phone 250 383 6864 (toll-free 1 888 232 4444)
fax 250 383 6804; email to orders@trafford.com
Book sales in Europe:
Trafford Publishing (UK) Limited, 9 Park End Street, 2nd Floor
Oxford, UK OX1 1HH UNITED KINGDOM
phone +44 (0)1865 722 113 (local rate 0845 230 9601)
facsimile +44 (0)1865 722 868; info.uk@trafford.com
Order online at:
trafford.com/06-2939

10 9 8 7 6 5 4

Other books by Pete Sarsfield

Running with the Caribou (Turnstone Press 1997)
Hollow Water (Turnstone Press 2000)
Suspended—travels close to home (Pottersfield Press 2003)

recent comments:

"What I like best about his work is that he comes to so few conclusions. In a structured world, it's refreshing to see someone who isn't convinced of the rigidity of things, who is, instead, open to the shifting perceptions that come with moving from one place to another."

- Linda Turk, in Thunder Bay's *Chronicle-Journal*

"I thoroughly enjoyed reading your stories in *Hollow Water*. I'm glad I picked you, as the storyteller for my Budapest-Prague train ride, over Dostoyevsky. Thanks for the smiles and the occasional lumps in my throat."

- postcard written from Prague, writer unknown

"How has a Canadian writer with as clean a prose style as Pete Sarsfield's avoided our notice? I'm in search of *Running with the Caribou* and *Hollow Water*, his two previous small-press books, after reading this integrated patchwork [*Suspended—travels close to home*] of measured but atmospheric pieces concerning various Canadian localities, large and small, from Grand Manan Island in the east to Mayne Island in the west."

- George Fetherling, in *Vancouver Sun*

for Jan   *for Sarah*

Pete Sarsfield

for Fr. Charles Hurkes

Bob Jeffery

Contents

Horse's Ass

Masters Us

"... I glimpsed the flux
of what exists and does not exist
a wavering between disappointment and joy
and knew there was only a moment left
before the little gap in time healed itself..."

- Al Purdy,
in *The Woman on the Shore*

Introductions

*I*collect images, mere glimpses. These are snapshots at dusk without a flash, distance views without a telephoto. My favourites are the blurred ones, only hinting at context and connection.

A simple idea has nibbled at me over the last few decades, at least I *think* the idea is simple, an ordinary thought, but maybe it is profound and finely twisted. (Who knows these things; who could judge?) The idea is this: occasionally we achieve a clearer and deeper look at the centre of a person, a concept, or an event than would have been possible if we were intimate, too thickly loaded with history and expectations.

This goes against our learned sense, our current societal reliance on data and experts and painstaking proof. It smacks of a return to visions and powerful intuition. We are uncomfortable with things deducted this quickly, especially if we are the ones labelled as magic or witch, or are prone to falling in love. The truths of reason and science hold dominant position over the truths of feeling, for a while at least, as we near the end of this number-haunted era. Later, when the pendulum catches its swinging breath, we will revert; we always have.

In spite of this, and always when least anticipated, such as on a sidewalk passing or in a stranger-filled city and looking out a window while happily alone, the sudden view reveals the heart of the matter. Or, so it seems.

My method of dealing with this clash of truths fits well with our wildly ambivalent time, in that I simply qualify the idea. I cope with these glimpses by assuming that they are rare, a random fluke, the rubbing together of chance and chemistry to gain a spark. I'm off the hook; spontaneous combustion *does* happen, but not often.

On a round table in a room where I now spend part of my life is a long wooden kaleidoscope, a gift that offers patterns of intricate order or chaos by peering squinting into the peep-hole end. Whether one sees order or chaos is a matter of feeling, and it varies from person to person, and for some from day to day. It does seem to be consistent that most are fascinated by the patterns, for a while, held still by their beauty and their (non)sense.

Pete Sarsfield
Kenora, Ontario
2006

Glimpses speak to me. They whisper, shout, giggle or call out for my attention. It happens everywhere and occasionally I catch them with my camera. The photographic glimpses in this collection were captured over almost 30 years. Selecting these images during a cold bright winter weekend became an engaging and personal process. A picture is worth a thousand words and for me each of these images tells a story. Pete's stories and the images co-exist in this volume and give you the opportunity to consider our glimpses and potentially create your own. Enjoy.

Bob Jeffery
Sudbury, Ontario
2006

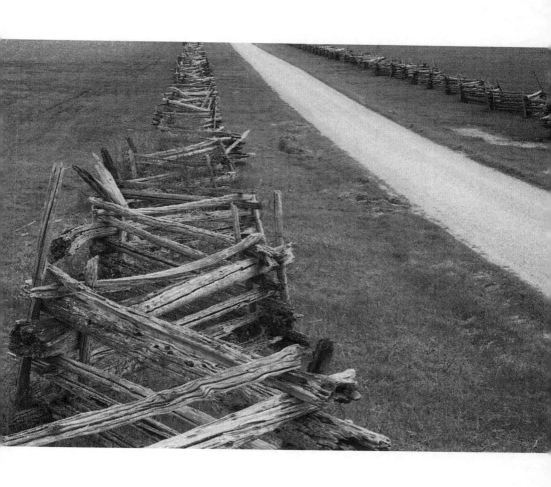

Exploring Manitoulin Island on a sunny weekend afternoon thinking about the people that built the fence and farmed the land. -BJ

Hideout

"We live in all we seek.
The hidden shows up in
too-plain sight. It lives
captive on the face of the
obvious—the people, events,
and things of the day—to
which we ...have long
since become oblivious.
What a hideout ..."

- Annie Dillard,
in *For the Time Being*

"Absolute truths hide in our simplest habits."

- John Ralston Saul,
in *Voltaire's Bastards*

At 6:00 a.m. on a January morning...

At 6:00 a.m. on a January morning, with a full moon easing down over the east end of Kenora's Coney Island, near where the Narrows widen to become the Lake of the Woods, a man comes off the island and onto the walking bridge that connects to the Lakeside part of the town.

He is carrying something on his shoulders and is pulling a loaded sled, moving from shadow to light between the six lights spaced along the narrow walkway. There are railings; he is safe.

The man plows through the mist that is rising from the small patch of rapid open water; then he's gone from sight.

It's a mid-winter Saturday evening...

*I*t's a mid-winter Saturday evening at the main-floor bar of the waterfront hotel in Sault Ste. Marie, and I'm exploring the concept of dark beer. Most of the three hundred delegates have gone home from our three-day meeting, and it is cold out there in the world, blowing a snowy gale, so the bar is almost empty. Earlier in the afternoon, I experienced a brief and uncharacteristic spasm of image-seeking cultural solidarity, leading to my wrapping in sub-arctic gear of hat and great-coat and mitts and boots, then leaning and wading into the wind and snow to get to the nearby palace of theatres. I rarely indulge in cultural solidarity, as I find the alternating forced camaraderie and interpersonal mayhem to be harmful to the unfolding of the routine sweet serenity of my day. Some noxious influences are more palatable when bottled.

The gods obviously agree with my biases, as they so often do, and mid-way through a barren and depressing movie, the theatre's fire alarms erupt and we are quickly ushered out into the snow. I nod a humble thank-you to the gale and trot home to room #306, where I change from my arctic explorer outfit into classy stool-sitting gear. This permits a retreat to the bar, where I'm resigned to drown my disappointment.

I perch in a comfortable high-backed chair with Saturday's *Globe & Mail* to hand, order Upper Canada Dark and ask if I may eat at the bar. No problem; I'm given a menu. The TV over the bar has Hockey Night in Canada going, sound low but loud enough to hear. The background music for the whole place is subtle jazz, Stan Getz-like. There is one other person sitting at the bar, and he's a hockey fan, not a talker. The bartender is friendly and also willing to leave me to my paper. I'm a winner, holding a full house.

When she brings my seafood pasta, the bartender sees me abandon the *Globe* and we settle in for some standard mid-winter blowing-snow hockey chatter. She knows what she's talking about, and I don't, so I say just enough to keep it going. She asks if I know there is a game in town tonight, right here in St. Mary's River city. I tell her I didn't know and I'm not moving, and she agrees to take this as a compliment. I am a potential financial bonanza, after all.

For a careless instant I forget our shared hockey history, (more movies might help), and ask about graduates from The Sault to the NHL. I ask who has made it. She looks at me, deadpan, then dips her head and inquires if I've ever heard of Wayne Gretzky. Oops, of course, G for Gretzky, Great, and Greyhounds. I ask if she watched him play here. She had a season ticket then and wasn't working so many nights, so she saw The Great One play many times. I ask if you could tell. Were you able to see what was coming? "You could tell he was good, very good," she said, "but he's not very big. There was no way to know what was going to happen. We just watched and went home. We didn't know we were seeing history." Then, she paused. "I don't go much, anymore."

We make a shared unspoken decision to not go down that particular fork on the avenue of angst, instead moving back to our own unfolding and unrecognized legendary moments. I ask for another Upper Canada Dark. She nods.

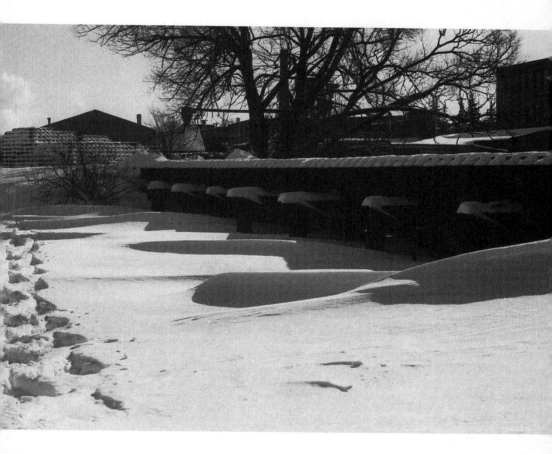

Walked this bridge to classes at Waterloo. A bridge to a brighter future. -BJ

I'm sitting in the empty living room...

I'm sitting in the empty living room of the Recovery Home of a First Nation in northwestern Ontario. I have a deep need for a coffee, but I'm alone and feeling shy so have plunked my ass down without looking around. I am mugless.

It felt like home the minute I drove onto the Reserve, even though I'm an alien, a non-Anishnabe, "a damn white-bearded *doctor*, for god's sake" is how one aboriginal acquaintance put it recently, as if that explained everything, especially the bad things.

When I drove into town, I waved down a pickup coming toward me and asked, "Where is the Treatment Centre?" I was directed, appropriately, to the Band Office, which I should have known enough to do on my own without behaving like an idiot tourist by interrupting a small truck's trip. At the Band Council building, I introduced myself, explained my purpose, and was then and only then directed to the vulnerable and, therefore, protected Recovery Home, down a few buildings on Anishnabe Way. I'm ever alert for dislocation-level leg-pulling in aboriginal country, especially when I've made no discernable effort to be thoughtful or sensitive. I'm ripe for the Anishnabe Way plucking. However, it appears that the street name is deadpan serious, so I open the door to leave. "And it doesn't have a sign," she calls after me. I look back; she, too, is deadpan.

After pulling into someone's yard and receiving directions and a smile when I declared I was lost, as if that required saying, I find the Recovery Home, which as advertised has no sign. I park off to a side and enter the bungalow building. There are voices coming from out back, but there's no one near the entry door in what looks like a Zeller's Living Room; it looks almost like that. The room has the standard bulky patterned chair and couch, and then off to the side another twin couch as a bonus, as well as a big, heavy, wooden, coffee table and a symbolically marooned, disconnected footstool. There's also a photocopier and a fax machine, possibly useful in breaking the Zeller's pact of conformity. I remind myself to avoid anthropomorphizing other people's furniture. I need a coffee, strong and soon.

A woman comes into the combination living room and communications centre, glances at me, nods, and keeps walking. I say that I'm here for a meeting. She stops, nods an "ok," and then goes on through an arch to the connected kitchen, where she pulls down a mug and advances on a moderately large coffee pot. I ask if I can have one, too. She smiles, indicating wordlessly that I didn't need to ask. I take a mug labelled with ORANGEVILLE BRAMPTON STRATFORD NEWMARKET OTTAWA, figuring who would care if I used *that* one. I fill it to the brim with hot, strong coffee and then sit back down to watch the room and to wait.

People come and go; some speak or nod to me, and some do not. I'm visiting a country where one tries to neither question or direct, and where one watches and waits. I'm at home in spite of my many differences, but I'm the only one here who knows it, and even then there's a possibility that I'm fooling myself. That, too, is acceptable.

From a living room just off the kitchen...

From a living room just off the kitchen, in the Musquodobit Valley of Nova Scotia, a friend writes:

"The morning of May 4th was gray and mild, warm enough to work with neither jacket nor shirt over my t-shirt but cool enough that my sweatband did not begin to drip while I forked six loads of manure into the spreader. I was able to hitch Lady and Marlise to the machine with no help, and no trouble worth calling trouble. Between trips to the hayland, while I was forking, the team stood perfectly. Usually, when I'm training a horse to the job, I tie the lines to the spokes and hub of a front wheel so the lines will automatically tighten on the bits if the horses try to leave. With the first two loads that I forked while the team was hitched, I just laid the lines on the ground, which is to say on the muck near the manure pile. Thereafter I hung them on Lady's hames, lest I further soil my hands. I was confident I knew the nature of my partners in this work and that my trust was not foolishly placed. That proved to be correct.

With delight, I minded the kildeers' and flickers' sounds while I was forking. Things were going so well that I was surprised by my reaction to the chittering of swallows, the season's first and earlier than usual. I was surprised because I thought I was already about as high as I get. Upon hearing the blessed swallows, I stopped forking and looked overhead, hoping they were not flying so high as to be invisible. They weren't. There were three. They flew over me, heading north. Something swelled in my chest. I almost burst, almost sobbed with joy. Perhaps tears welled up with that overpowering feeling of loving welcome.

Kathryn says I cried when Masa was born. She makes up stories, so I doubt I should take her word over my recollection that I laughed with delight. But maybe there were tears that she misunderstood. You may be able to settle the issue. You were there, too. I must ask you, sometime."

Lionel tells the story...

L ionel tells the story of a kitten who had become damaged beyond hope and, as a result, was wild and dangerous.

It is Sunday afternoon, and there are fourteen people gathered in a wandering circle in the open living area of an image-filled, hexagonal, green-shingled house on a sloping field just off the Appin Road in the Bonshaw Hills of central Prince Edward Island. Some of us know each other, and some don't. Most are curious about each other, and a few are also cautious. Two are from South America and are left quietly alone, because of the wall of language; it seems there's nothing to be done about this, at least not by any of us.

We've all eaten and talked in small food-based groups, and now we're reaching the end of the afternoon. We're coming up close to some genuine issues, even the prickly edges. One of the exchanges considers whether men, cursed as we are by our violent and oppressive history, are ever capable of sane and caring interaction, of being trusted with anyone's future.

Lionel defuses a tense moment by telling us about this kitten he knew, and he does the telling with a humourous off-hand grace. The animal had experienced some frightening accident, being locked for a lengthy while in a dark and foodless cellar or some such. This had twisted it, and it would strike out at anyone who approached. The cat was now beyond all reach.

A friend came to visit, and he recognized the harm that was there in the kitten, and even more importantly, he decided to help. For a whole weekend he persisted in carrying the kitten wherever he went, carefully, inside the front of his jacket, contained but free enough to see and move. The healer did this even though the kitten (and it has to be imagined that the animal was small, bearable) would bite and scratch, terrified, angry, desperate. This is how I heard the story, how I pictured and embellished it, as Lionel was using flexible calming words to paint the scene, making the inner elaboration easy and possibly even honest. By the end of the chest-and-jacket weekend, the kitten was less wild, as the terror and brutality had been eased. It had been given a chance.

We soon leave and go several different ways, and we are once again comfortable and possibly connected. Lionel has denied that his story was allegorical. He made this claim with a self-effacing smile.

A stranger died...

A stranger died recently. He lived next door to me, but I only met him once, in the hallway, when he was being helped to move furniture. He had already been living there for several weeks, but he said that he'd been camping on the floor all that time. He grinned at me, with eye contact, when he told his helping friend that I wrote things. He didn't volunteer that he liked the pieces, and I didn't ask. We spoke only two other times.

At night, late, if I'd be getting home from some trip, or more often just unable to sleep at 3:00 a.m. and wandering about, I'd see his apartment lights on, with the curtains open. My bathroom and his living room gave angled views of corners, probably only rarely glanced at, too private for scrutiny. There was never a sound from his area, but then we had only one small shared wall. Our apartment entry doors were side by side in the hallway, and there's a common laundry in the basement, but we didn't run into each other, not ever. Occasionally, there would be something hanging from his doorknob, and as I'd enter my place, I might hear his radio, but that's all—next-door neighbours and strangers.

A few months ago he phoned me in the evening to ask if I knew of anyone who would be able to give him advice and medication for a longtime problem. I asked for a few details, trying to avoid prying but needing enough information to know how to proceed and who to recommend. This is a town where it is very difficult to get a family doctor if you're new to the place, but the next morning I related to a local physician what I had interpreted as a cry for help. The doctor readily agreed to be available at noon, on his lunch break. I called the home number my neighbour had given me, to tell him of the appointment, but a recording said the number was disconnected. The telephone information person gave me a totally different number, and I phoned this several times but got an answering machine each time. My neighbour finally called back but said that the noon-hour appointment would be awkward for him, as he had some things he had to get done. I stated clearly, firmly and also close to pleading that seeing the physician was the wise thing to do, and he eventually agreed. I have no idea if the appointment was kept.

About ten days after this exchange, my neighbour was found dead in his apartment. I heard about this on a Sunday evening, when there was a fire in my fireplace and CBC radio was playing Bach. The patterns of both were somewhat comforting.

Over the years, a couple of my relatives and friends have made similar last-ditch appeals, and for similar reasons. For them, too, it is obvious to me that I could have done much more—visited, phoned, left a note, anything and many things.

On a memorable radio interview, I heard a Buddhist monk offer the opinion that it does not matter if a person is a Buddhist, all that matters is if that person has a good heart. I wonder what my stranger neighbour would have thought of that, at 3:00 a.m., if I had cared enough to ask.

I've just finished supper with...

I've just finished supper with a friendly acquaintance, at a restaurant on Harbord St. in downtown Toronto, just off Bathurst in the area called the Annex. My plane had been late getting in and it was lashing rain at the airport, plus I'd been up and going since about 5:00 a.m., so when I stumbled from the cab and onto the crowded restaurant patio it was late and I was mute with tiredness.

The person waiting had a table saved and hadn't minded the wait. My luggage was easy to stow, the rain had now stopped, the evening was washed and warm, and the people on the covered patio seemed to be enjoying themselves. My dinner companion acknowledged my fatigue and carried us through the evening with kindness, cleverly. This was one of those don't-worry-things-work-out evenings that are maybe self-fulfilling prophecies or the result of an atypical resolve to go with the flow instead of against it. It needed to be carefully noted, so I did.

After dinner we exchanged a spontaneous good-to-see-you-again hug and went our ways. I waved at a cab out on Harbord St., and when I climbed in, the sweet smell of pot was thick. The driver said, "I'll leave the windows open to air us out, it being a warm evening and all; ok?" and he smiled into the back seat at me. "That's great," I said. He was about my age, with an accent I think of as middle European, wearing glasses, balding, and with a medium-length gray-haired pony-tail. I asked if he knew who won the Jays game. "Just finished listening to it," he said, "and they only lost 7 to 4; only left 12 men on." He had a warm and relaxed tone, not too sarcastic, and we talked back and forth about the Jays' troubled pitching and about the elusive necessity of a winning attitude and the related ability to believe in one's ability.

For a few seconds I considered trying to adopt his amused and accepting approach to vicarious defeats, before deciding that I've become quite attached to my more usual confrontational, judgmental, ironic, no-quarter-given-but-lots-asked style. To each their own, I thought, in the back seat of the comfortable open-windowed cab.

The music on the radio snapped me out of this self-evaluative pre-funk, as it was excellent mellow jazz, not my standard cab fare, not even at 11:00 p.m. near Queen's Park in the centre of this tiny perfect universe. I said, "Great choice of music; Ross Porter?"

"Yeah; I switch back and forth in the evenings between him and 91.1 where they do a mix of jazz and classical. What do you like?"

By this time we're ambling south on University, approaching the turn into Gerrard, a street that reminds me of my daughter Sarah, every time. "I listen a lot to quiet jazz and some classical," I said, "but I know absolutely *nothing* about any of it. I'm on the outside looking in, with no understanding of the mechanics or the subtleties."

He glanced back at me and nodded and then said, "That's not my problem," reaching over to his radio to switch away from CBC to the 91.1 station. "Hear that?" he said as a classical piano piece came in. "Know who it is?"

"Not a clue," I answered.

"It's Liszt. All you have to do is listen more, and more carefully, and you'll get it. Who *do* you like?"

"Bach, very much, especially the shorter tone-poem things, the fugues and Goldberg Variations, all of that."

"Oh, sure, that's good; but why not try to branch out to Liszt and Chopin?"

"It sounds as if you have a full life," I said to him as we pulled up to the Delta Chelsea's Gerrard Street entrance, "what with baseball and a skilled ear and warm evenings with fresh air and all." He grinned and said, "Life *is* good, is it not? Here's home for you, for tonight. Listen to more Liszt; don't forget."

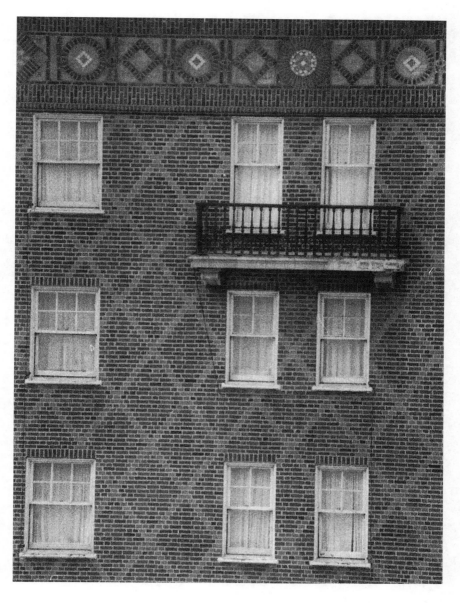

Looking out of a hotel room in St. Louis, I wondered if the people living there know or appreciate the patterns on their building; then I realize, I don't know what my hotel looks like. I smile realizing self discovery is the last insight. -BJ

A small chocolate bar is passed…

A small chocolate bar is passed to me on a Toronto-to-Winnipeg flight, a "snack" as the time of day and the airline budget doesn't permit anything more substantial. I look at the bar, fix on it, and the flight attendant and the person jammed into the middle seat beside me glance over, both strangers and both curious; am I about to make a fuss?

Not at all, at least not out loud. I'm far too mature for that, and maybe even too resigned, nostalgic, and lonely for lost friends. I'm going to just sit back and eat the bar.

As I unwrap it I'm remembering a person who was a friend of my heart and her fondness for these bars, some years ago. She would eat a lot of them, and since she was a skilled enthusiast, she could turn a piece of chocolate fluff into something special and unique, a symbol of spontaneous outlaw happiness, a gift to be shared.

She could achieve this alchemy with many things: with snowshoe trails through a huge stand of upright burned-over dead spruce, or helping someone become less terrified of their serious illness by sharing her warmth and humour, and always by treating each day and each person with gentle respect.

We were dancing in another person's crowded basement room one night, both moderately drunk, with the music very loud, when she stopped moving to look me in the face and tell me she loved me. I knew this and felt the same way, and I deeply hoped she wouldn't mind that she had spoken clearly during an unanticipated pause between songs from Fleetwood Mac's RUMOURS album. We never knew who heard, and I never cared.

On the plane, the man in the middle seat beside me grins and asks if I enjoyed my meal. "Very satisfying," I reply. He scans my face, looking for irony but not finding it.

On a bright Winnipeg summer...

O n a bright Winnipeg summer morning, a man in his thirties and a boy about age five are carrying things, walking from an apartment building toward a large rental truck. The boy is holding a small cardboard box, top open, while the man is loaded down with a lamp, some clothes and curtains over his shoulders, and some other loose things, hangers and round mailing tubes under his arms. The boy looks uncertain, tentative, and the man in his ball cap, sweatsuit and beard looks beyond weary. He is lost, whipped.

He juggles the underarm things and then deposits the lamp and everything else up onto the high back of the truck; some of them are semi-flung. Then he places the boy's box on the truck, more carefully, with not a word between them all this time.

The boy points at the back-of-truck lift platform and says, "Can I ride on it?" The man barely glances at him, doesn't answer, and starts to walk back toward the apartment building. After taking about three steps, he stops, turns around, comes back to the truck and says, "Sure;

hop on," and then reaches for the switch. The boy smiles at him, a huge and direct smile, then stands on the platform, holding on, ready to go.

It's the first evening...

I t's the first evening of the four-day Winnipeg Folk Festival, at
about 5:00 p.m., and the early comers are lined up to be the first
to get their tarps in place for Main Stage. Benita and I are early
comers. Ben is the one with the tarp, which in her view is all-too-rare
evidence of the universe unfolding as it should. She is off with the
other elite holders of numbered squares of pink paper, allowing them
to secure a privileged spot near the stage. No running allowed. I'm
with a gaggle of others back behind the orange rope, watching the tarp
unfold.

A woman standing beside me, a stranger, says, "Excuse me? What
are we doing? Are we supposed to wait here while they do something?"
I explain the walking of the tarps and our behind-the-rope role of
combined cheering section and (im)patient watcher whilst the Head
of the Tarp secures our rectangular place. She looks at me, more or less
for the first time. I look at her, more or less for the first time. She is
in her mid-twenties I'm guessing, short and fit and round, with blond
hair, blue eyes and huge tattoos over most of her arms and shoulders,

coloured ones, intricate, spiralling connections of images and designs. She either senses my approval or doesn't care a whit, but either way she answers my questions. She keeps those blue eyes aimed directly at my face. Her tattoos are spectacular. Her left arm has a complex web of red, blue and black flower-like weavings, an instant personal favourite.

She has come here from Toronto, and she mentions the world's irrational fear of unusual respiratory illness in that city, to her scorn. So far we're on the same page. She rode a motorcycle here, and she tells me the make and identifying number. I haven't a clue. It isn't a Harley. I nod my sage recognition. She smiles, knowing I haven't a clue. She loved the long run around Lake Superior, as I do, but found the stretch from Thunder Bay to Dryden "a bit long."

"God finds that stretch a bit long," I opine. She grins. I ask if 59 is too old to learn to drive a bike, "preferably without killing myself." She gives me an emphatic "No, it is not!" and tells me what to do and not do, the dangers of weather and people, and which of my own attitudes to avoid. "At first you'll be freaked by the ground going by so fast, even if you're only going 100. It all seems to be so fast and so right *there*, because it *is*. You have to learn to relax, but not too much."

She drove alone from Toronto and was charmed when a man stopped to ask if everything was alright when she had pulled over for a rest. "That wouldn't happen in most places, or if it did, you wouldn't want it to, you wouldn't let it. Here, it was ok." It's her first Winnipeg Folk Festival, and she's up for it.

Motorcycles and tattoos are dangerous, and I work in the danger-prevention business. If this decorated solo bike rider were my daughter, how would I feel? I easily decide that I'd be fully proud of her, in much the same way and for many of the same reasons that I am proud of my daughters. It's a complex weave, all the patterns, all of our rides.

Another friend spots me and comes over. The motorcycle rider goes quiet and drifts away, instantly, and there's nothing to be done. I occasionally look for her over the weekend, when I remember, but we're always in different places.

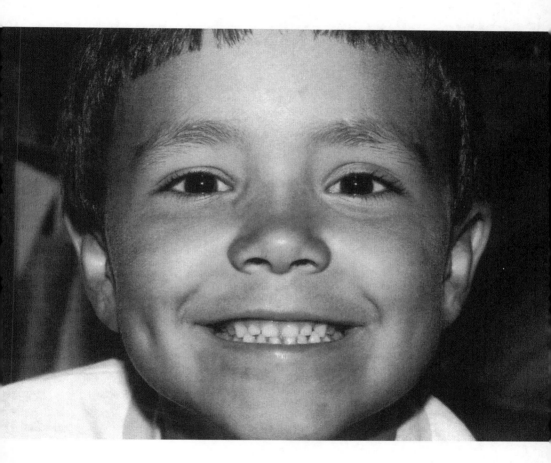

Darren smiles. -BJ

As I drive the rock-cut roads...

A s I drive the rock-cut roads of northwestern Ontario, I listen to CBC radio, habitually and playfully. (One can play the radio, just as with a musical instrument, if one wants to take the time and make the effort. My theory is that this playful opportunity also applies to airplane and bus travel, elevator encounters with strangers, middle-of-the-night insomnia, doing laundry at 9:00 p.m., and responding to answering machines. All these mundane activities of daily living are prime instrument-rehearsal times, and we need to practice.)

On this mid-afternoon summer weekday, I'm on the road between Kenora and Fort Frances, near Nestor Falls, and the highway is awash with Americans driving huge sport utility vehicles and lugging boats behind, at high speed, into what they must see as a sparsely populated northern wilderness. Every second tree has a police car idling behind it. I decide to let our ever-so-impatient Yankee cousins support our legal system and highway construction fund. I slow down to just barely over the 80 km/hr speed limit. The drivers of the SUVs whipping by me at between 100 and 120 km/hr give me harsh or puzzled looks, which imply I'm a menace and deranged beyond hope. What a price is paid for serene survival, a familiar Public Health theme.

Bill Richardson is on the radio with his *Roundup* show, sharing his clever, gentle, ironic, "sad goat" self. He asks us to inspect our persons for "totems," those symbolic items we wear or carry to remind us of cherished and inherited connections, and/or to bring us luck. I'm always willing to accept direction from Bill Richardson, so I mentally conduct the suggested review of self. I am carrying these mythic symbols, on this day I am:

• In my left pants pocket, there is a pewter humpback whale inside a pewter oval. It dives as far as it can bear and inspects what it finds there, and it *always* has to surface for air. I often hold this whale, or put it out on the table in front of me, when I need to share my daughters' space.

• In the right pants pocket, I have a small oval beige stone, on which there is a painted image representing *health*. The paint is fading; the sentiment is not. It helps keep me healthy, if I am willing to accept it.

• On my right wrist, I have a woven friendship bracelet, mailed from Mexico, wide and bright and warm in blue, yellow, green, and a few splashes of white. It reminds me of a friendship and a relationship about which I have no need for reminders, the way totems are meant to.

• On my left wrist is another cloth bracelet, from Alberta or Manitoba, (I'll have to remember to ask), slim and vivid in red, yellow, blue, green, with edges of black. I have taught myself to try not to expect gifts of friendship and also to practice the stillness as well as the dance, and this gift was (I think) a kind response to my making gradual progress. It was also a hug.

• Around my neck is a carving made from found antler. It shows a long-faced, balding, bearded man, and it has a character carved into the side, encouraging serenity. I view this etched face, tattooed for peace, as a step along the unending continuum, from acceptance to rejection and back again, over and over, until it all goes back to antler.

• Also around my neck, to add balance, is a silver whale's tail. I would be seaweed to the whale, anytime and for all my time, and this diving tail may help.

• My small finger, left hand, has a silver ring, made by a member of the Salish Nation and bought in BC, with a raven carved into the circle.

I wear the markings of whale, raven, friendship, and the rune of calm, as well as the sites of absence. If I were from a family clan system, there would be fewer choices, in some ways, but my family doesn't adhere to clans, so I can adopt myself into several systems of myth. The myths sustain us, but only when we have taken full care to choose the supportive ones.

A *recent Gemini Awards presentation...*

A recent Gemini Awards presentation of statues, which I was watching on CBC television from a hotel room near the middle of some trip, named a once-familiar person as one of the members of the winning group. I leaned forward, in room #121 of La Place Rendez-Vous in Fort Frances, and tried to spot a face I hadn't seen in fifteen years. He didn't get near the microphone or the camera, leading me to smile as I imagined him choosing instead to stand back and just watch it all unfold, including his own designated role.

I first met Nigel over 25 years ago, on a resolutely anachronistic medical ship that was used for a tuberculosis X-ray survey on the northern Labrador coast. He had talked his way onto the ship and the two-month survey, using his self-effacing shy wit and charm, and a promise to give the Grenfell Mission "free" copies of all photographs, to get the hitch-hiking spot on this unique trip. He needed a vehicle, but his vision was already clear.

It was instructive to watch Nigel work, and I've often tried to imitate the patience and generosity of his methods. In the morning he'd come out on the deck of the STRATHCONA, which had anchored for the night in a sheltered harbour, and he'd do a slow circling tour of the ship, scanning, looking for textures and themes, trying to find the angle of the day. He usually did not have his cameras with him on this first circle scan. It soon became apparent, but gently, that he did not want to interact with anyone during this time. He'd have much preferred to be invisible; just looking, thanks.

Nigel didn't accept that his photographs could be "art." He did see, if I understood him, the necessity of being responsible, careful, in his expropriation of images. He was aware of the dangers inherent in the capturing of stories, and he worked to respect the reality of other people's moments.

Sitting in room #121, I agreed with Nigel, yet again, that you can find depth wherever you look, even at the Gemini's. I'd allow Nigel to steal my image anytime, or at least I'd try to surrender to it, but only after he carefully circled my life's decks.

I'm in the midst...

I'm in the midst of a relatively calm small-room, closed-door discussion, in Fort Frances, Ontario, regarding the benefits and risks associated with immunization, and we're pretty much in agreement; this is a no-heat interaction. As a result of this welcomed harmony, I'm in a low-adrenalin state, which allows me to mentally drift, to indulge yet again in a stolen absence.

This one takes me back to the 1950s in Nova Scotia, when the vaccine against polio was being introduced. I was in grade 5, and my sister Sue was in grade 3. The whole school was lined-up at the community hall, and one by one we rolled up our sleeves and accepted the needle, upper arm. Very little was explained to us, no questions tolerated, the usual medical noblesse oblige. I remember the weather as cloudy, windy and cold, leaves off the trees, no snow on the ground. I have no idea if this part is accurate or if it's just another cumulative rolling fiction of recall.

What I *am* sure of is that when I got home that day my mother asked me about the needle. As I told her of the community hall scene, and she was the first one to encourage me to paint all such descriptions in full and vivid colours and strokes, my mother started to cry. There were several very good reasons for her to cry on a regular basis, but she rarely did, being smart and tough and not given to remorse or pity, self-directed or otherwise. I was shocked to see my mother cry for no apparent reason and asked what was wrong. She said it was about the polio shot. I told her that it hadn't hurt *that* much, really, it hadn't. She wiped her eyes and laughed and said hell no, that wasn't it, explaining that the tears were because she was so happy that Sue and I were no longer at risk for polio. I wasn't up to speed on either the spectre of polio or the concept of tears-of-happiness, so my mother told me that a couple of her school friends had died and been crippled by the disease, and she was relieved that her children wouldn't have to face this. The tears were dried, vanished, by the time she finished telling me about her lost friends.

My mother died before the next school year started, so looking back I can see why she may have been relieved—one thing she no longer needed to worry about.

The radio is on in a hotel room...

The radio is on in a hotel room in Dryden. It's late evening, and I've got paperwork scattered around the table, so in reality I'm only half listening to the radio and half concentrating on the memo-mess. (And as Yogi Berra would say, with the *other* half I'm just drifting around somewhere altogether different.) An aboriginal person is well into being interviewed on the thoughtful radio show, but he hesitates in the opening stages of an explanatory story. He breaks the flow. The CBC interviewer doesn't get it, so he pushes, asking why the hesitation? The man explains; he can't use the story; he doesn't own it, ". . . it's not my story..." He's embarrassed, and I'm guessing it's not because of the bump in the smooth unfolding of the *IDEAS* program but because he came close to a real breach of conduct; he almost forgot himself. He names the owner of the story, in effect saying if you want to hear this, ask the one who knows, not me.

The CBC interviewer and I are from the same culture, or so I assume based on his name and speech, and I think I understand his confusion and frustration, but I've also lived in and near First Nations communities for much of my adult life and, as a result, have a flicker of recognition of the significance of "the story." Aboriginal stories and songs seem to be the equivalent of Euro-Canadian family histories and societal codes and identifiers, all the dates and names and traceable numbers, very personal and very potent. The stories and songs an aboriginal person has are the signposts to the meaning of that life, and they are not to be tampered with.

The exchange ends quickly as they both seem to shrug and move on, stepping back from the canyon edge of cultural differences.

The Innu duo Kashtin sing, in one of their early songs, "I'm a brown-skinned man; that's what I am." There's so much and so little in those words; culture and gender, reality and risk. Maybe, just maybe, if we recognize our differences and treat them with affectionate respect, we'll be able to just step across the canyon's gap, if we're invited and if we care to.

I'm a story stealer but cannot work up even a faint lather of guilt on that account. We're fair game out here, every one of us with our intricate, contradictory, hopeful, and revealing stories. We're all free theatre; that's my culture, and I'd better be careful.

I'm in Sioux Lookout for several days...

I'm in Sioux Lookout for several days of meetings, staying in a log building that is in the midst of tall pine, spruce and birch. The building has an attractive dark-red tin roof, and within hours it feels like home. I ask questions and am told that this building, and other similar ones nearby, are occasionally available for rent over the winter months, at a remarkably affordable cost. This availability and affordability occurs because of capitalistic necessity, when the affluent tourists thin out.

For the three days that I'm in the building, I think about this possibility of a new home, a temporary winter home between my anticipated summer living on BC's Gulf Islands, Nova Scotia's Cape Split, and also in L'Anse au Clair, Labrador, and Dawson City, in Yukon. As a result, there are occasional mental drifts away from the meeting, allowing me to plan where I'll put rugs and paintings in this huge cabin, how to soften the lighting, where the dining table will have the best view, whether Bach or Van Morrison will dominate the music selection, who will be permitted to visit and who will not, and whether or not I'll have a telephone or a car or two cats. One of the highlights of the three days, and there are several, is the sound of full rain on the dark-red tin roof. It is a reassuring beat.

When the meeting is over, most people leave in the usual manner and in the usual rush. I get to stay in town, for yet another meeting the next day. (For now, for a while longer, meetings dominate my life. This will not be allowed to persist.) In the late afternoon I go out on Sioux Lookout's new walking path, which extends all the way to the Frog Rapids bridge, over five kilometres from town. This is a wonderful path, wide and adequately removed from the highway, rising and falling with the land, both adapting and following, an independent connection.

There are very few people on the path on this chilly October afternoon, and we nod as we meet and pass, sometimes saying 'hello' and smiling, sometimes not. A group of four, seeming to be a family, is slowly walking ahead of me, and just before I catch up, they veer off and cross the highway to a street of houses, where lights are on in the late-afternoon dusk. As they turn off the path, one of them acknowledges my nearness, waving hello and goodbye. Ravens fly overhead, calling. Cars and trucks noise by on the main highway, captured by wheels and speed. It quickly becomes night. I turn back.

I've left a light on in my rented place, and as I approach the dark yard, I stop to look at the lit window. It appears to be warm, like a home.

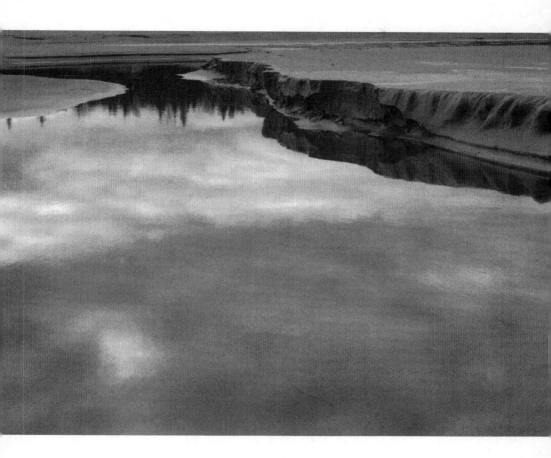

Perspective can be tricky; I see a large river with high bluffs, not the small spring stream carving its way to Lake Huron. -BJ

Early on a November weekend evening...

Early on a November weekend evening in a companionable Winnipeg apartment, there is a *Dallas* reunion on television. The actors who portrayed JR, Sue Ellen, Bobby, Pam, Lucy, Cliff, and Ray in the 1970s and 1980s are seated on stools on a stage, facing an audience and answering preselected questions, accompanied by big-screen replays. The "top ten cliffhangers" are counted down, and filmed blunders and pranks are "seen for the first time." The actors not only look older, the twenty years having been typically effective, but some also appear subdued and defensive. There are several central *Dallas* characters not represented or mentioned, because of death in some cases and perhaps because of time-better-spent or ongoing feuds in others. The reunion is strained and contrived, tackiness elevated to an art form, which is entirely appropriate for *Dallas*. I completely enjoyed the show all through its run, and I now watch every instant of this return to gleeful trash, again transfixed.

The personal and the general have intricate and captivating cross-border connections, even when it comes to the comedy of culture. Watching the stage-bound *Dallas* actors attempting one more turn to this particular over-the-top tune, another stage is recalled. On the south Labrador coast twenty-five years ago, the medical work was done by resident nurses, supported by Nursing Station staff and a maintenance man who doubled as a guide for overland trips, with occasional peripheral input from a travelling physician. There were no airstrips or roads, just small float- and ski-planes, boats, and snowmobiles, and there was minimal television or radio reception in many of the villages. We were much better off, but very few of us knew it. (Those of us who did know, usually the "outsiders," were sometimes semi-amiably referred to as "spies;" the judgement contained a degree of sense.)

Several times a year, we would go from Charlottetown, a town of 400 people midway along the south coast, to Norman Bay, a village of 40 to 50 people, where we'd do a one- or two-day medical clinic. We three—nurse, guide and doc—would travel the approximately 50 kilometres on three snowmobiles in winter, towing komatik sleds piled with equipment and boxes of drugs and charts, or in one small open and loaded boat in summer. We always looked forward to these trips, as they seemed to represent a key reason for being in Labrador.

Norman Bay was one of the few tiny communities on the coast to survive the "resettlement" spasm of Joey Smallwood, a couple of decades before. When the school and the Post Office and all other government-largesse services were removed, as had been promised for any places refusing to capitulate and shift to a larger community, the Norman Bay crowd just stayed put and kept fishing. (I'm told they are still there, even though the fish are not.)

One Friday night in the late 1970s, we hadn't finished our clinic and so had to stay over. We were usually able to manipulate our activities so that we were obliged to overnight, allowing us to enjoy bunking wherever offered, with the shared meals and talk. As it was a Friday night, we were also going to be able to share *Dallas*.

There was no electricity in the village, another government plug pulled or never inserted, but one of the homes had both a gas-powered generator and a small-screen TV. About fifteen of us gathered in the tiny living room, sitting close to the television on chairs and floor and with a few standing, all to enhance the view of JR's sneer. We were remarkably quiet for the entire hour of snowy flickering alien drama. Southfork, Texas, came to Norman Bay, Labrador, and both were improved.

Later, after the show and the post-game analysis had ended and the generator had been turned off, I picked my dark-path way back to this night's home, again noticing the striking absence of light pollution along this part of the Labrador coast.

I've miscalculated...

I've miscalculated weather and roads, leading to a white-knuckle, radio-off, full-focus, mid-December drive from Dryden to Kenora in blowing snow and icy curves. Before going home, I need to visit the grocery store, having been on the addictive highway for most of the last two weeks. In the parking lot, as I ease out of the car, I stop to stretch and loosen, glancing by reflex at the nearby hotel. A few windows are lighted for guests, or to create that impression, and the sign on the top is bright, even in the snow.

Buildings have associations with people and events; otherwise, they are flirting with being bare of meaning, even when beautiful, perhaps especially when beautiful. This round hotel beside and over the water and ice in Kenora, for instance, is my daughter Jan's, in my mind. When it loses that connection, it becomes a superbly situated but calculating and chilled monument of plastic.

Jan worked there for a summer several years ago, and I enjoyed walking down the hill from my apartment to meet her after the front-desk shift was over. I'd take a back route, along a lane behind three houses that face the harbour, then on a walking path sloping down through a clump of trees to another lane, coming out beside the hotel, more or less. Jan and I understood each other, and it was summer warm with conversation and connection, with boats in the harbour that seemed non-intrusive and mobile, with acceptable intentions. Everything combined to give a mere building the virtue of context.

The hotel is dramatic, multisided with a straight-edged portion for each tier of rooms rising, making an angular circle. It is built over the water, to a large degree, leading in summer to the sound of waves underneath as you walk on wood slats beside the front sidewalk or along the paved parking area in the back, itself linked by stairs and ramp to a floating or ice-bound dock. There is a main floor with entry space, meeting rooms and a front desk; eight floors of guest rooms, many of which face the Lake of the Woods; a top-knot of dining room, kitchen and exercise areas; and a tall, bright-red, four-sided sign proclaiming **INN**, all topped by side-by-side, equal-sized flags, one American and one Canadian.

Without the connection, there is only cool distance, even if next door. This hotel is at risk of becoming just another lonely impersonal and alarmingly necessary place to visit when I'd rather be somewhere else. They need a large **J** on their roof.

The concept and reality of home...

The concept and reality of home evolves in layers, along with the view from eyes of the beholder. The two, concept and view, appear to be linked and even interdependent. Van Morrison acknowledges that "home is where you hang your hat...," and then slyly adds, ". . . but you'd better check it out first." In order to become comfortable in your own skin, it seems useful, maybe necessary, to be comfortable in the room where that skin finds itself. One of the many rooms where I look up to find myself is in the hotel, over and again, at least a hundred days a year for decades in a row. Turning this into a homey experience requires effort, preferably not of the self-pitying or lying-to-self kinds but instead of the rearranging-reality kind.

On checking into Toronto's downtown Delta Chelsea at mid-afternoon on this occasion, I immediately rearrange room #2560's easily moveable furniture to fit my mental map, a longstanding reflex similar to a dog marking territory. (We are cousins.) Then, I amble down to the Market Garden cafeteria, through comfortable sounds and along familiar hallways and personal eccentric routes. I talk with Vicky at the cash register, after we have smiled recognitions and shaken hands and I have waited for the tourists to pass on by. We volley back and forth about our kids and the hotel business and our different workplaces' shared paranoia regarding all things infectious. Vicky contributes intelligence, warmth, and calm courtesy to my recurrent self-service Toronto dining experience.

On leaving the cafeteria, I go to the flower shop in the lobby, where the owner recognizes me as "the Kenora guy who sends flowers to his daughters." I could do much worse than to have *that* painted on my inevitable urn of ashes. We talk, and I buy.

After changing into workout gear in my room, the hotel reinspection leads to the fitness place on the 26th floor, where I again try to convince myself that painful sweating is joyous. The manager of the facility asks how I've been. The place is nearly empty. We agree that many people seem to feel that avoiding exercise will prevent viral infections. We are not amused and don't bother to pretend. I continue to sweat, and he folds more towels.

I get up early the next morning. The meeting I'm here for can't begin until 10:00 a.m. because lawyers are involved and it has become evident that they are sensitive and fragile creatures, not about to be pushed to any brink by precipitous starts. I, on the other ledge, am a physician and so have been up and going since 5:00 a.m., saving whole communities of lives and polishing a novel in between. At 9:00 a.m. the housekeeping person knocks and asks if she can make up my room. I haven't met her before and, therefore, assume she must be new here. We talk, and it turns out she is not new.

Sylvia is from a village in rural northern Portugal, near the Spanish border in the Porto district. I acknowledge a passing acquaintance with the fine liquids of the region; she smiles. Sylvia's mother died when she was five years old, and she was then sent to an orphanage in Lisbon, where she lived until she was fifteen. It became her home, and the people were her family. Her recollection is that the orphanage was a kind and helpful place, with caring people and an excellent education. She traces directly to the orphanage her present strength and independent spirit as well as her ability to work, as they insisted on the children earning their way through daily contributions of productive effort. I go fishing for negativity, but Sylvia tells me that the work was not unduly difficult. It was appropriate for a child her age, she says, helping her learn enduring good habits. She is not surprised or offended by my question. She has thought about this and has recognized others' reflex assumptions.

Sylvia was married at age seventeen, "almost twenty-five years ago," she tells me, with a direct grin. She likes Canada, it is her home, and she is connected for life to Portugal, also her home. "You have two homes," I say. "You are wise." "Yes," she says, and we share another smile. "Me, too," I say, giving room #2560 an embracing arm-sweep gesture. I thank her for the place to hang my hat. She nods acceptance; she knows.

From a small, blue house...

From a small, blue house near the Hillsborough River in PEI, a friend writes:

"Today, when I got home, I put up some Christmas lights—I've done it only once, and then I think I used duct tape. This time, because I feel like I am 'home,' I bought little doohickeys at Canadian Tire and did the job RIGHT! I hammered my thumb and froze my fingers but thankfully didn't break any bulbs. So, I have one string of blue lights in a rectangle around the top opening of the 'fence' on my veranda. After I did that, I put two sets of mini-lights, (one white and one red, because that's what I had), in a big mayonnaise jar, plugged them in and put them on the table by the window. It's sparkly and surreal.

While I was doing the outside lights, the sun was setting, and the finale was one of those sunsets that's only visible on the horizon, with dense gray cloud above it. The earth was outlined in red, and I could hear a noisy crowd of geese who were arguing about whether to leave tonight or get a good night's sleep, followed by a hearty breakfast and set off for the south tomorrow! Then I put all the house lights off, went out the back door and walked down to the road without looking back, and then turned to survey my place. It looked lovely; all worth it!

This may be my first adult Christmas not putting up my own special tree. Almost-strangers ask me if I'm going to hang my tree again this year and will it have candles on it. The decorations are almost all homemade, and almost all are red or white. It reflects me, and even though I won't need to do it this time, I enjoy the thought."

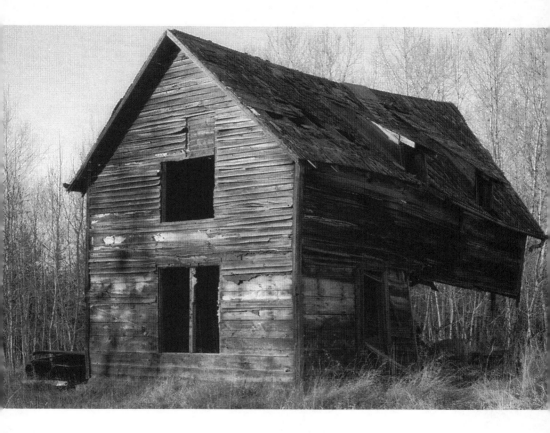

A house without a corner stone, standing…for years. -BJ

Horse's Ass

" 'No reason to get excited,'
the thief he kindly spoke.
'There are many here among us
who feel that life is but a joke.
But you and I, we've been through that,
and this is not our fate.
So, let us not talk falsely now,
the hour is getting late.' "

- Bob Dylan,
in "All Along the Watchtower,"
from *John Wesley Harding*

We're involved in an interminable...

We're involved in an interminable, convoluted, multi-voiced discussion regarding the "need" for name tags for Public Health staff. This brings up several interesting issues, including whether it makes public servants vulnerable to public rage by having their last, and therefore traceable, name exposed to scrutiny and whether name tags are useful only in urban areas, where no one knows anyone else nor do they want to. Conclusions are elusive. It's at times like these, and there are many, that I have the urge to run screaming from the room, fleeing the bureaucratic toxic fog, perhaps choosing to fling myself in the path of a low-flying flock of seagulls. This is not a useful urge and definitely is not career-enhancing. Therefore, I retreat into my own self-generated inner-fog and dredge up full recall of another name tag episode, years before.

A past friend, then nursing in the hospital at St. Anthony, Newfoundland, and later at a Nursing Station along the south Labrador coast, was taken aside by the rigid-backed, sphincter-clenched Head

Nurse, a British Matron, and told that she really *must* wear a bra, as ". . . the doctors already have enough to think about." My friend was so taken aback by this observation and demand that she was speechless, a wildly uncommon occurrence for her. The Matron, sensing a vulnerable moment with a usually obstreperous nurse, galloped even further into behaviour-change mode, adding, "I must also insist, and this is vitally important, that you wear a name tag at all times." The Matron then whisked off down the hospital corridor, leaving the nurse standing, open-mouthed and fuming.

The following day my friend was on the ward again, still without a bra but now sporting a brand-new name tag. The Matron came along, peered briefly at the name tag, ignoring the rest of the chest, and said, "Ah, nurse, that is *so* much better," and off she went, smiling, her authority verified and secure. As well as being content in her bureaucratic bliss, she was also, it appears, in need of glasses, as she'd failed to see that the name tag read **YOU HORSE'S ASS**.

I veer back to the foggy meeting, feeling calmer, already planning what *my* name tag is going to say.

Many of my signposts…

Many of my signposts come from old rock songs. Accept your truths from wherever you can find them is my motto, one of a shifting many. (Consider yourself blessed if you can find truths anywhere at all; there's another one.) For example, Randy Newman once lamented in song that "*. . . maybe I'm doing it wrong…*," without ever specifying what it is. Along the same line of thought, Neil Young has introspected out loud:

"*. . . thinking about what a friend had said. Hoping it was a lie.*"

My conclusions are bordering on straightforward. Our friends shouldn't lie to us, unless we insist and are willing to risk the friendship, and they must help us do it right, some of it anyway, some of the time. I'm increasingly convinced that, if strangers felt similar obligations, our signposts and our journey might become friendlier.

I recently did a presentation to a group of strangers, with a few friendly acquaintances sprinkled throughout. The subsequent anonymous written evaluations indicate that maybe I'm doing it wrong.

glimpse – Pete Sarsfield

My approach to presentations, which has evolved over thirty years and owes much to the story-telling examples of aboriginal people, is to link stories and ideas from writers and from personal experiences, so as to offer different-angle views of the topic being discussed. The linkages are always loose, fluid and occasionally obscure, and all of this is on purpose. Truths are in the ears and hearts of the beholders, and my job is to get the people in the seats up off their third buttock, mentally speaking. It is to be expected that the resulting connections and conclusions will be wildly different from person to person, as they should and must be. This wide range of responses is usually welcomed, at least by me.

There are times, however, when the spread of reactions leads me to wonder if we are all just too different to even try to share this space and perhaps we must focus more fully on merely staying away from each other.

On the typed summary of comments sent to me by the conference organizers were the following:

- *"self-indulgent unfocused ramble;"*
- *"information too personal;"*
- *". . . if we only had people like you in government...thanks for your comments;"*
- *"excellent...I really enjoyed the presentation...you had my full attention;"*
- *"the points were lost in the anecdotes and I got nothing I could run with conceptually or otherwise."*

On they go like this, from opposite ends of the response continuum with the middle bare, including our collective navel. I was forced to return to Randy Newman and probably not for the last time. If people so strongly like *and* dislike what I'm doing and if the aim is to get through to most of the people most of the time, as we are so clearly encouraged and expected to do, then it might be wiser and easier to just stay safe and dry.

Dry and safe, safe and dry; there's a chant to live by, if one is dedicated to offending as few as possible, other than oneself, of course.

All will be clarified in any eventual final evaluation. For *that* one, I may be holding my breath.

In the past eleven years...

In the past eleven years, I've driven the Kenora-Winnipeg highway hundreds of times, using it as the best route to and from the Winnipeg airport, or to visit people I care for, and to do such necessary urban chores as digging for hidden partial truths in a medical school library. It is a two-hour stretch of highway that I enjoy and respect. I view it with such intense familiarity that it is tempting to feel that I could drive it without effort, as if I am so aware of every impending curve, speed trap and rock-cut that I don't need to bother paying full attention. This would be a dangerous illusion, making me vulnerable to the suicidal night deer at Falcon Lake or to the obligatory idiot passing on a blind hill anywhere at all. This stretch of highway helps me to remember the quick-change relationship between ease and chaos, a useful reminder.

It isn't always tragedy that reminds us of this relationship. Recently, for instance, I stopped for gas at the Petro-Canada station on the eastern edge of Winnipeg. The pumps were busy, with cars behind and ahead of me, so I quickly filled the tank, ignored the dirty windshield, and hustled in to the pay-up counter. I had a full bladder, so I asked the bored and harassed cashier, "Can I leave the car there for just a minute while I hit the bathroom?" "Ok," he said. "But don't be too long."

I hurried to the back of the station, and on entering the multi-person washroom, I did a quick scan for the urinals, but on not instantly seeing them, I went into a stall instead. This was distress mode, and there was no time for exploration. The washroom was empty. As I was assuming the customary standing-male pre-voiding position, I heard people entering the washroom, talking as they came. I froze, just prior to sphincter relaxation, as the voices were female. I rapidly dropped pants and sat on the toilet, with my large male shoes tucked out of sight to the centre, and tried to urinate with a hopefully reassuring wide-spray splatter. More women came in, occupying the stalls on either side of me and with more at the sinks. Some were talking, and some were not. I hoped that women exhibited the same terse dedication to duty and avoidance of chatter to strangers as do men in this situation. I also hoped that my car didn't get towed and that no one would shout at me when I eventually had to leave.

After several minutes, the washroom finally emptied, so I got up and out in a fully-zipped flash, deciding without hesitation to skip handwashing this one time, Public Health be damned.

As I went quickly across the now two-acre-wide store, I avoided looking at anyone, although I was sure that I could feel the stares and glares. I had my ". . . partial sex change…" defense ready to go before I hit the door but didn't need it, as the Social Taboo Police didn't catch me. I was relieved, so to speak, because they are intense when they get rolling.

See what I mean? Chaos and ease, side by side, just a narrow stall away.

The theory is...

The theory is, at least according to *AS IT HAPPENS* on CBC Radio #1, that a man listens by using only half his brain, thereby eliminating either the abstract poetic tangential-leaping portion of the mind or the organized literal methodical half. The author of this study on brain wave patterns has concluded that women use two sides, men only one. "And, so, what's new in *that*," asks the host, who coincidentally is a woman. I take offense; indeed, I do. Well, the male author replies, it could be that men need only half a brain to do the whole job. Some more-or-less good-natured lobs and volleys then ensue, across the gender netting. I switch to *DISC DRIVE* on CBC #2, which I get late on a cable-feed from BC and which at that very moment has on a wailing *Romeo and Juliet* excerpt. I switch to silence.

My cell phone rings in the other room. It's 7:45 p.m., I'm at home with a plainly listed number for the normal phone, and I do hate this additional and intrusive phone-monstrosity, *but* it might be one of my daughters calling in from either Calgary or Florida to rescue me from parental angst, so I leap to answer.

"Who's this?" says male-voice buddy.

"Who are you looking for?" I say.

"Brian!" he responds, quick as a communicatory flash.

"Nope. Not him; you got Pete."

"Who the hell's '*Pete*'?" he says, and I can hear a grin in embryo stage.

"We *don't* want to start a relationship here; we really don't. You've got the wrong number," I say, but I've got on my *no-sweat* tone.

"What number *is* this?" he asks. We are both definitely listening, with our whole brains, all four aggregate sides just whipping along, the literal wrong-number parts and the having-fun-through-playful-error parts. (Where is a researcher when you really need one?)

I tell him my number.

"No, that's not what I hit, not what I *meant* to hit, anyway. Sorry, bro.," he says and then adds, "Take good care," and he smiles; I can hear the smile.

"You, too. Glad we got to talk," I say, and we hang up, none the worse for wear. I liked being called "bro." I notice this as I hit the cell-phone END button.

If I sent the transcript of our two-strangers wrong-number call to *AS IT HAPPENS*, would they listen to it, with all their sides? I think I'll leave them to wallow in unilateral bliss. I switch back to CBC #2, where they're playing Bach this time—much more like it, very two-sided.

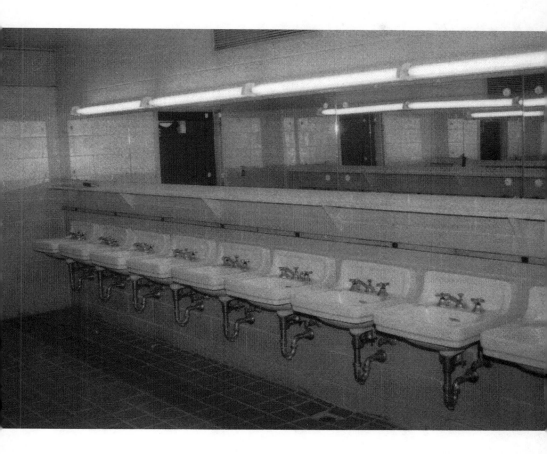

I felt like an individual when I brushed my teeth at these sinks, 2nd from the end was my favourite, but 20 years later, I only see structured depersonalization. -BJ

Some of the wisest, funniest...

ome of the wisest, funniest, most capable people I know do not like to eat alone in public places. These people are women.

Most tell me, when I ask, that they rarely sit alone in a hotel dining room and they insist that they are treated differently than a man would be if he were eating alone, especially in the evening. They say that they receive scrutiny and condescension and are often placed at one of the worst tables, somewhere back by the kitchen or the serving station. Verbs are always revealing, and I used "they insist" and "they say" because I was initially sceptical. As well as naïve insensitivity contributing to my scepticism, the origins also included simple, open-mouthed incredulity, since these people are intellectually and emotionally tough and profound. They are people I listen to, with care. Hell, I pay attention when they breathe, and so I didn't want to believe their version of their dining lives. It offended me, on their behalf.

Recently, I spent a weekend in Whitehorse, Yukon, and it was a nostalgic, stimulating, frustrating, challenging, and ultimately futile, three-day, kaleidoscopic weekend. I ate alone a few times and was pleased to do so, as it gave me the welcome solitude to ponder the telling absence of imaginative progressiveness in so many health-care bureaucrats.

For one of my solitary meals, I arrived early to the nearly empty hotel dining room. I was immediately shown to a table and had my order taken and caffeine level repeatedly attended to, all with no fuss and yet with an adequate exchange of pleasantries so that we could both keep our Canadian citizenship intact. "Lunch for one?" leading to "Yes, thanks; no smoke; lots of coffee"—that sort of polite semi-ritualistic blather.

About 20 minutes later, a woman came in alone, approximately my age, and dressed much as I was, in casual chic. She paused at the entry door and then waited. The server eventually came over and said, "For lunch?"

"Yes, thanks," the women said.

"Just for one, or will someone be joining you?"

"No, just me; non-smoking, please."

"Just one? You're by yourself?" the waiter asked, and she wasn't moving toward a table.

I put down my coffee cup and started taking notes, eyes down, ears up. "Yes, *just me*, for lunch, non-smoking, *please*," the women replied, with eye contact and a whole new edge to it now, much quicker to notice and to take offence than I would have been, up to that day at least, or until the power pendulum swings the other way. The server, herself a woman and herself alone, showed the diner to a table next to mine. There was a possibility that there would not be a 20% tip coming from either table.

The diner and I chatted across the aisle about flying, weather and food, but we stayed well clear of the ongoing travails of solitary dining. I'd like to think that my overwhelming charm, or my fulminating humility, helped reduce her personal pissed-off level, but I don't extend that to any hope of a reduction in the societal gender-bias situation. Unfortunately, realism occasionally intrudes into my wishful thinking.

On that note, I owe a specific apology to some friends. This is it.

I'm out for an end-of-day walk...

I'm out for an end-of-day walk, and I would like to get tired. It has been a featureless day, empty of either conflict or a sense of joy, and my home is a hotel. The sidewalk leads me along.

A man comes out of a house just up ahead of me, carrying a piled-high clothes hamper and a large box of laundry detergent. He crosses the sidewalk in front of me without glancing my way and opens the back door of a small car. A woman comes whipping out of the same house, moving fast toward the man and the car, and says loudly, "You're taking my soap, too? I can't believe you! You take my money and the car **and** the soap. You are *unbelievable*!" She walks up to him, standing very close, and grabs the box of detergent, which as luck would have it is the one with the bright rainbow on the cover. The man stands beside the car, looking at the ground. The women goes back toward the house, moving more slowly.

I keep walking, not missing a step. I'm feeling very tired.

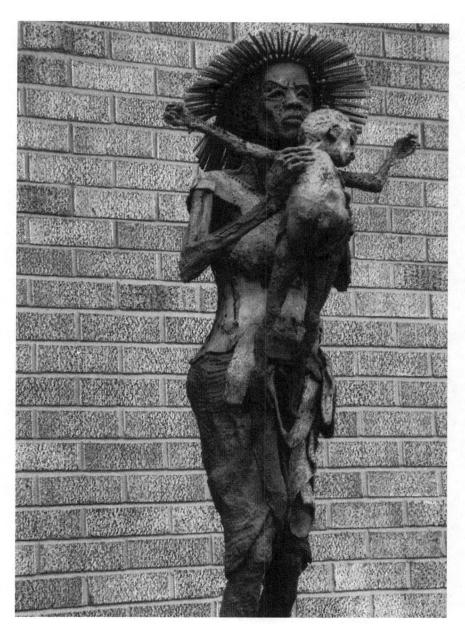

The Vietnam war memorial statue is difficult to look at. I found myself captured and repulsed by its image. -BJ

Two of us, friends...

Two of us, friends, are walking on a side street during a late summer day that is hot but not overwhelming. The older trees provide the sidewalks with an arch of shade. My friend stops walking and says, "look," pointing between houses. I do look, but I don't see what she's pointing at, so she says, gently, "Just *look* at the angles and shades." I adjust, focusing as she intends, as we wish we could all the time, on the gallery of the day.

Where my friend has pointed, there are varied and overlapping tones of colour and shades of light, angles of fences and shrubs and lawn, framed by the two side-by-side house walls, all of it with rich, full-leafed trees as its backdrop. She is right; it is there, and all I had to do was be open to actually *seeing*. My friend smiles as I confess to walking around blinkered.

What I *don't* confess to, fearing loss, is the fact that she has surprised me. I hadn't known that she had that type of vision—a painter's eye; it hadn't even occurred to me. I was doubly blind.

As we walk along, quieter and even more connected, I wonder if she was smiling at one or two insights.

A colleague was flying from...

A colleague was flying from Winnipeg to Toronto and so was I. We both lived in Kenora and worked together in northwestern Ontario, so we usually knew where the other one was or was going. This time we didn't know and surprised each other by showing up separately in Winnipeg for the same mid-day flight. We sat together and tried to not talk about work but mostly failed. We'd had some heated debates over the two years of working together, but usually these didn't matter.

We landed in Toronto, on time, talked out, comfortable with our shared space, and ready to go to work. We were going to different meetings in different parts of the city, and my friend was renting a car. I was about to get a taxi or bus into the city centre, but she offered me a ride, saying it wasn't far out of her way, and she also said that it would give her a chance to drive in the city.

This person is a city person and was finding northwestern Ontario to be non-urban and lonely beyond bearing. She was homesick for the city, and this was one of our differences that we had decided to just let be. She actually *wanted* to drive me downtown, into the heart of the claustrophobic chaos and risk that is inherent in any large city, or so I see it. I mentally shook my head in disbelief as I happily accepted the offer.

We got in her rental car, and on our way out of the airport she cut a guy off, badly, no excuse. He blasted the horn, truly angry, as it had been a fairly close call, and he then saluted us with his middle finger. My friend fingered right back, grinning but not with the embarrassed "oh damn, oh shit" grin you'd expect in that situation, not at all. She was grinning the real joy-filled thing. She was ecstatic. The offended driver looked at her as if she was berserk and then just waved us on, with no real heat or malice in the motion.

After a discrete minute or so, I asked about the origins of the spontaneous joy I'd just been lucky enough to witness and survive. She said, "God! I just got the finger; *already*! It feels so *good* to be home!" and she was practically skipping as she drove. I sat back, buckled in, vowing to take a very large bus into town next time.

Aliens are demonstrably different. It's fortunate that we're kept in different locations.

I'm sharing these pieces...

I'm sharing these pieces with a person I once knew and still respect, wonderintg out loud if it is possible to capture the extraordinary depths that are hidden in glimpses of the seemingly ordinary. More to the painful point, I'm wondering if it is possible for *me* to do so.

I'm asked, "Am I in any of these?" and it wasn't the question I was looking for. I have no idea if it would be better if my answer were 'yes' or 'no'. My grasp of the obvious and of the depths buried in plain view suddenly becomes suspect to me and perhaps to others as well.

I ask, "Do you *want* to be? I thought I'd go for anonymity and ambiguity, the display of shadowy figures on the edge of the lit stage, that sort of thing. Am I wrong?"

"I don't know which I'd rather; I just wondered. It doesn't matter."

I think that perhaps I need to adjust my radar, but I keep the thought to myself.

We're in the Koocheching County...

We're in the Koocheching County Law Enforcement Centre Training Room in International Falls, Minnesota, just across the Rainy River from Fort Frances, Ontario. There are twenty-two people in this windowless, concrete-walled basement room—twelve Americans and ten Canadians. I work with one of these people, herself Canadian, and she has sent me a pre-meeting note that instructs, "we are <u>observers</u>, and we're <u>not</u> to talk, especially <u>you</u>!"

The agenda uses Roman numerals, but these Americans appear remarkably un-Roman, approaching being friendly and gentle. I'm assuming all virtue is due to their northern location and associated proximity to humble Canadians. We are the conquered-but-assimilative colony to the Neo-Roman Empire, and they seem amazingly good-natured about it.

Within five minutes of our self-introductions, I'm asked for my opinion. I adopt my internationally famous laconic and self-effacing attitude, and inform the Chair and hushed participants that I've been told by she-who-demands-obedience—(gesture to my right, toward sinking Canadian)—that I must shut-the-hell-up. The Chair exerts authority, and I'm given permission to speak. (I'll pay for this, irrevocably, but it's worth it. I reject laconic, vociferously.)

The meeting is focused on potential cross-border terrorist attacks. I have difficulty imagining the random forces of worldwide evil becoming proud of themselves through damage to the municipalities of International Falls and Fort Frances, but I have recently been informed that I'm naive about the gradual and pervasive progression of evil and that I am inclined to ignore feet in the door of the slippery slope. Glancing around at my position in the grandeur of the Training Room, I begin to understand the logic of the slippery-slope theory and silently vow to immediately begin work on increasing my paranoia.

As well as being ever vigilant to recognize and stop the viciously demented true believers in our midst, however, perhaps we need to also work on our concern regarding the destructive casual villains already active, ones which include ourselves. We show no signs of easing back. These ongoing threats range from poverty, racial and gender-based harshness, unforgiving stereotypes of several types (see above), smoking, guns, alcohol and various other drugs, and above all the increasingly dense swirling fog of environmental destructiveness. I suggest this international view to the Training Room.

The Chair intervenes and calls for a vote regarding my initial *shut-the-hell-up* directive, nodding in new appreciation to my colleague. The vote in favour of the edict is unanimous, including my own. I sit back to take notes, laconically.

Walking toward the plane...

Walking toward the plane, leaving a northern community when I'd rather stay, I'm crossing the gravel skirt of the runway, moving away from the terminal building, already weary from the prospect of movement to come. The plane will take us south, and I'd much rather that it got safely lost and took us in the other direction. I'm lonely for the north.

A man I'd once treated for urinary calculi, "kidney stones," years ago in another place when I was a family doc, comes out the door after us and hands me an inch-wide rough-edged stone-like object, stating that he has just passed this and thought I'd like to have it as a souvenir. He gives me the "stone" and a farewell pat on the arm, and then goes back into the terminal.

The Flight Attendant has overhead this, as we were walking to the plane quite close to each other, and she says, "That *really* must have hurt!" Grateful for the relief from the awkward sadness of leaving, I grin at her and explain that possibly buddy is trying to deceive us about both the stone *and* the size of the chute required to pass such a thing. I then show her that this is, in fact, a rock from the airstrip. She laughs, and later smiles whenever our eyes meet, as we fly to the other country in the south.

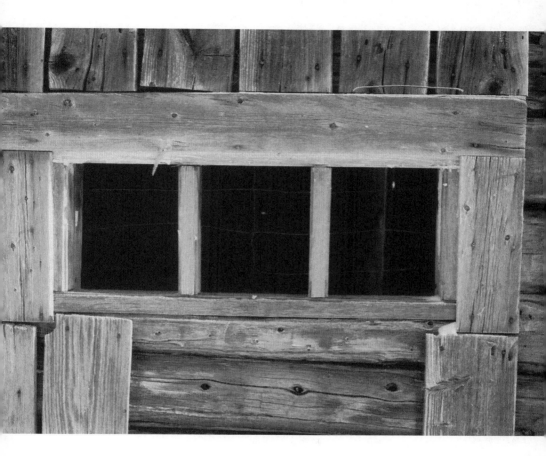

A window fenced from the inside. The contrast of weathered wood, wire and handy man carpentry fits the back woods location this house was found. -BJ

A middle-aged, white guy...

A middle-aged, white guy is eating a muffin, bran with raisins it looks like, and he's drinking orange juice, at one of the small tables scattered about near the fast-food stand at this semi-northern airport. (I'm not talking about myself here; this is another middle-aged, white guy.)

This airport sells many bags and boxes filled with food to be taken further north for those who are starved for high-fat, high-sugar, low-nutrition, kill-you-deeply-dead-but-it's-worth-it snack food. When I lived in Cambridge Bay, then in the Northwest Territories and now in Nunavut, it was fried chicken that was most prized and often lugged cold and congealing from Yellowknife to the northern "hamlets." Our culture exports exotic appetites.

The person I'm watching is a sub-species classic, one of the diminishing numbers that will soon be placed on the endangered list but which is as yet nowhere near extinction. He is dressed in creased pants and a crisp open-necked shirt, with a v-neck sweater and a suit-jacket over, and has a huge parka stashed in the chair beside him. He has on big boots, and I'll bet there is a big warm hat and big thick mitts to match. He is a hired advisor of some kind, no question. This is a person who makes a living directing northern people on the affairs of their lives, over and over, year after year, on and on. His crowd has made itself become essential.

A while ago, the numbers of these advisors were indeed out of control, threatening the environment in their dominance and fouling their own nests because of their single-mindedness.

A thinning-out, a culling, an energetic harvesting, has been long overdue. It must be asked, however, if we really want to see this species vanish altogether from our lives? I think not. A few of them (of *us* that should be, I admit it) should be allowed to survive, chattering and strutting the fading plumage, always pretending to be ever-so-clever. Without advisors, who would humour the day? We need consultants, not for counsel, absolutely not, but instead for sheer entertainment value. They are as sustaining as fast food, and we should keep some around—only a few, though, just a few.

My daughters...

My daughters were dancers. Sarah lived in Toronto for three years while going to Ryerson, and Jan was at the University of Calgary. As a result, I occasionally got to wander around those campuses, getting a feel for the hallways, bookstores, student centres, and cafeterias, all the places that formed the backdrop for those days of their lives. I received few ageist glances. Maybe I was mistaken for a professor, but more likely no one noticed or cared. This was comforting.

One morning at the University of Calgary, in the food-court area, I saw a young man wearing an old-fashioned baseball jacket, with a heavy flannel middle part and leather sleeves, knit collar and cuffs, and several crests and labels.

I used to have one of those. Even though I couldn't play worth a damn, I went to all the practices and tried hard all the time, so while the bench was my permanent position I wore the team jacket and felt that I'd earned it.

The juxtaposition of the university hallways and the ball jacket triggered a flashback labeled "18th Century Literature," from Acadia University, 35 years ago. I'd been putting considerable effort into this course and was getting nothing beyond mediocre results, so I had requested an office chat with the prof., to discuss my writing and her marking, and to find out about dismissive comments she had penciled in the margins of my papers. "What's going on here?" was the question at the heart of this meeting. The professor, all sphincters apparently in full and ever-lasting spasm, admitted quite freely, casually even, that she was unable to give me an A in any part of the course, essay or exam, because I wore a baseball jacket to class "not just once or twice but *every day*" and so could not be taken seriously.

I remember her use of the word "unable" regarding the marking of my work, and my subsequent suggestion that perhaps she meant "unwilling." Now the patronizing academic gloves were off, although my recollection is that she never did let her syntax slip from its lofty perch of well-punctuated and complete sentences. I was told that I might have a certain facility with language, but this was glibness, not depth, and it most certainly was *not* erudition, so perhaps I should run along and read some Hemingway.

There was even an uncharacteristic flicker of direct eye contact during her brief verbal flurry, and I had to admit (to myself) that I liked her more than when I'd come into the room. She also had a point, not about the jacket but more painfully about the writing. I was at the beginning of a what-*am*-I-doing-here stage, (not for the last time), and the thought was also occurring to me that if she and similar others were my role models, I didn't want the role, not any part of it. So I advised her to root against the Yankees, always, no matter what the odds, and I left.

Would Hemingway, the self-doubting non-academic, have enjoyed the exchange? One can only wonder and hope. It certainly lightened my year.

A dancer writes from Calgary...

A dancer writes from Calgary:

"I had job training for catering last night. There was dance class and then rehearsals before the training, from 9:00 a.m. to 7:00 p.m., with a half-hour break at 2:30 p.m. I was late (they knew I would be) for the training, and it went until 10:00 p.m.

The training was ridiculous, partly because I've served in a restaurant before and this is a piece of cake in comparison, and partly because these people took three hours to deliver an hour's worth of material. For everything, every 'rule,' this woman had an example; '. . . this one time, we fired a girl for theft!'

Me: 'So, let me get this straight...you *can't* steal when you're at work?'

(Give me a break.)

I love the things like 'dress codes.' I know they're needed (I guess), but she was saying things like, '. . . black tights, *not* beige because then you start getting some girls wearing cream and some wearing white.' I was sitting there thinking, '. . . and *then* what happens? Someone wears red and all hell breaks loose? No one will know *what* to do. Where's the food; where are the guests? What kind of establishment is this? It'll be catering chaos!'

Then I calm down and think, 'This is a $6/hour job, so chill out. Everyone has to say these stupid things at the beginning.' You know?

I'll talk to you soon."

We are fourteen people seated...

We are fourteen people seated by role in the Patty Watt Room, on the west end of the third floor of the Design Exchange Building, at 234 Bay Street, in Toronto. The room has a high ceiling and white walls bare of art. It is square and large enough to hold a few tables and still give the required anti-intimacy spacing. There is no detectable inflow of air. Based on a passing scrutiny, the designers being celebrated, lamented or exchanged must have specialized in *ugly* linked to *sterile*. The setting fits the ritualistic morality-play process we are enduring. I admire the set director's appropriate sense of place.

We fourteen are adversaries, pseudo-judges and observers. Most of us are not impartial, and this includes the ones pledged to impartiality.

Occupations tell less about role assignment in this tight-lipped piece of expensive theatre than one might imagine or hope. There are six lawyers, a management consultant, a research physicist, two public health inspectors (one of whom doubles as an administrator, capable of switching roles in mid-sentence), a voluntary trustee, a transcriptionist, a bar owner, and a writer earning a living as a physician. As the drama unfolds, it becomes vividly apparent that the occupations indicate nothing about integrity, depth or honesty. While most of the fourteen actors already know this, the stark portrayal only increases our solemn dedication to pretence.

Three players have been sanctioned to adopt judge roles, designated a "tribunal" and seated at the front facing the adversaries and observers. These three pretenders have their own lawyer, seated at a separate, tiny table off to one side, never speaking, watching without announced reason. As two of the *let's-play-court* tribunal members are themselves lawyers, one has to hope for a potential infusion of expertise and adjudication at some level, but there is no evidence of this.

Oblivious passersby are talking loudly in the hall outside Patty Watt, leading to closure of large, double doors. The absence of ventilation now results in the room's air becoming even more deceased. This is a nice touch, subtle, barely noticed amidst the hypoxia. I make a note to congratulate the director.

The adversaries are relatively honest, a high point in the sewer, debating the limits of personal freedom when opposed to collective responsibility. (We are reminded through observation, however, that honest does not necessarily equal admirable.) The legal representatives of the opponents are amiable mercenaries who wear fine suits, speak in complete sentences, and exchange humorous barbs; there are no hard feelings; it's just a job. The observers and the genuine antagonists must be quiet, especially those most harmed by the process. The pseudo-judges stare straight ahead, blinking occasionally.

These three entrepreneurs playing at being judges are fascinating. They always arrive late and usually leave early, take long breaks for lunch or any other reason, all the while avoiding decisions or overt involvement. They are political appointees and are being paid on a perdiem basis. Whoever cast them should be exiled or praised, depending on your political bias. Perhaps that is the entire point—a Kafka-like satire mocking our pretentious lying games. We live and let others die through our art, here in the Design Exchange Building.

The actual Patty Watt lived from 1940 to 1995, and her life and work as a design pioneer are celebrated by a large plaque. If the gods are ironists they are cruel, as we have been warned, as the plaque's heading reads, "A Passionate Commitment to Excellence." A black-and-white and mostly grey photograph shows a woman facing the photographer, hands held loosely clasped in front and toward a shoulder. She has short hair, a direct gaze and a small, close-mouthed smile. She controls the camera.

I like Patty Watt's captured face and mentally apologize to this dead woman for the room, our pathetic roles and our society's uncaring greed, which has sanctioned the entire corrupt performance. I don't sense acceptance of the apology as the photo's unblinking eyes watch us through the weeks of our inept acting. "I'll be damned," I mutter, and someone glances my way.

After a day in Thunder Bay...

After a day in Thunder Bay discussing social equity, I have a craving for self-centered solitude. The nearby Valhalla Hotel jumps to the indulgent rescue, as the *All Inclusive Dinner Menu* features "Angels on Horseback" and "Pancetta Wrapped Cod Fish." Both are excellent, as is the service, the Canadian Pinot Noir, and the neighbouring tables' volume and content of interaction. All is good; social equity rules.

The server is quick and friendly, and she's interested in my praise of BC wine, Nova Scotian scallops and endangered fish wrapped in bacon. While she probably fully senses my absence of knowledge regarding the subtlety, focus or congruence of flavours (and anything else relating to the kitchen), she is generous and appears to inwardly shrug; it's a slow evening at Valhalla. She describes the apprentice chef, who prepared my meal, as being shy and insecure, by telling of his reluctance to accept praise. She'd like him to hear it in person.

She brings the chef from the kitchen to the dining area; backstage meets out-front, with both being uncomfortable with the encounter.

glimpse – Pete Sarsfield

He is quiet, but I wouldn't call it shy; definitions do vary. He is also a direct-gaze talker, young, calm, aboriginal, moderately certain of what he wants to be doing in five years (much more than me, I tell him, and he seems appropriately unimpressed). He appreciates the praise but not too much so, already knowing what he knows.

It appears that social equity comes in various guises. The Raspberry Crème Brûlée is ordered, with a sprinkling of almonds, to test the theory.

Masters Us

"We are not to know
why this and that masters us;
real life makes no reply,
only that it enraptures us
makes us familiar with it."

- Rainer Maria Rilke

"When we try to pick out anything
by itself, we find it hitched to
everything else in the universe."

- John Muir

Four of us are having a meal...

Four of us are having a meal at the TAP & GRILL on a Friday night in Winnipeg's Osborne Village. We are into the tap but not too much; it's balanced by the grill. We recognize and sometimes discuss this and other delicate balances. We are friends.

The restaurant is familiar, and it is noisy, full but not crowded, emotionally warm and also relaxed. Many people are animated, laughing and occasionally touching each other. There is no way to plan this; it has casually happened.

A woman at a nearby table, sitting with another woman, puts her feet up on one of the empty chairs, just for a few minutes. It isn't gauche; it's subtle, barely noticeable; she's at home.

The waiter smiles at us and seems to mean it. Another waiter, recognizing us from other days, nods and asks how we are. The music isn't too loud, and even though we'd prefer something more connected to the Mediterranean menu and general theme, (Ry Cooder in Cuba is my geographically incorrect vote), it doesn't matter; everything works, it all fits.

glimpse – Pete Sarsfield

At the next table are four women and two men. They are in their early to mid-twenties, not drinking much, talking in several shifting conversations at once, with much eye contact and touching. They are relaxed with themselves and with where they are. In the midst of an intense conversation between three of the women, who are all on one side of the rectangular table, one woman leans back and reaches over to begin to convert her friend's long loose blond hair into a pony-tail. The stylist has short dark hair. In the first instant of the hair manipulation, the blond woman raises an eyebrow, then smiles, and all three just continue talking; they've done this before.

The warmth and loud flow of the restaurant doesn't flicker as this intimacy takes place. Most diners and staff don't seem to notice, and those who have observed don't appear to be startled or quieted. The dark-haired stylist makes a jaunty side-of-the-head pony-tail for her blond friend and secures it with an elastic holder, all of this taking about a minute. They all keep talking, as do we, connecting; nothing is missed. The arrangement is suitable, balanced; it fits the evening.

When my daughters were
younger...

When my daughters were younger, they had a dragon-friend, *HISK*. (They may still be friends; I don't know.) *Hisk* recognized humans as primitive and dangerous, but she also felt that a few held potential, such as Sarah and Jan. As a result of her self-defined superiority, *Hisk* tended to be moralistic with my daughters, a tendency they ignored with practiced nonchalance. *Hisk's* only rule—a two-sided admonition with endless tangential variations—was (and hopefully still is) "be curious and be caring," a rule of balance.

During a book-talking at McNally-Robinson's store in Winnipeg, I suggest that a person writes out of curiosity, a private bearing-witness to one's own life, while publishing and selling the writing is, at its unusual best, a part of the caring or social-contract aspect of *Hisk's* one-rule. The two sides are necessarily linked, and they are different. At the book-selling, my articulation of this view was awkward and unclear, and I could sense *Hisk* rolling her swirling multi-coloured pupil-less eyes. I did, however, move some books.

I drive into Saskatoon two days later, scheduled to do another book-promoting session in a sibling bookstore. It's a cold snow-blowing mid-Saturday, and I know no one in Saskatoon. The person arranging my talk is setting up a podium and microphone in a corner of the restaurant as we jointly survey the landscape of empty tables. This isn't going to work; time for Plan B.

We agree to put me at a small table near the front entry door, with my books piled and displayed, an arresting presence, or so we hope.

At first, I feel silly and shy, vulnerable and exposed, sitting there as a charlatan used-word seller. *"Step right up folks; don't look away; have I got a deal for you. Words, words and even more words, ones to hang your soul on; they'll make you laugh and cry and roll your eyes, all for only twenty bucks."* Very few people stop. Twice, the front-desk staff take pity and make an announcement, "Near the front door, Pete Sarsfield is signing his new book...," and a few shoppers glance over before continuing in the other direction. Two of the restaurant staff, who had witnessed our setting-up-to-speak-to-silence performance, come out to see if I need a coffee or food, or sympathy. I accept the latter.

After about a half-hour, I get into the rhythm of the day, or to be more accurate I <u>force</u> myself to be observant, to be curious. The afternoon then relaxes and settles around me as I watch the building breathe and circulate. People move in and out in waves, with others circulating through the arteries of this large organism. The place is alive, conscious and purposeful. A few people do stop to talk, and this leads to walk-by listeners and copycat stoppers. We are a herd-animal species.

I sell four books in the three hours I sit at the table, and I'll remember all four:

• A woman and a man, together, are energetic travellers, and they are interested in my descriptions of places they have not visited. "Not yet," she says;

- Another shopper is primarily intrigued by the writer instead of the trips described. She looks me in the face and shakes my hand when she leaves, holding my book in her other hand;

- A man wearing a casual confident grin and a lock-eye gaze as well as a blond pony-tail describes himself as a "cultural geographer" and asks several relevant questions about person-in-place. I answer. He smiles, nods, and buys. I ask which part of my answer clinched the sale. He tells me without a flicker of hesitation and grins when I say that my answer was more luck than skill or truth. The sale isn't cancelled, but I'd like to think he considered it;

- The bookstore staff begin to display concern that I'll never leave, so I pretend to gather my stuff. Two people stop, a man and a woman, partners I'm guessing, and they have come out in today's blowing cold in search of ideas. They ask about mine, regarding curiosity and caring and writing. They are focusing on my replies and following the tangents where they may lead; they are actually listening—a rare occurrence. I like them. They buy a book.

I speculate, to myself, that things may be connected, some of them, some of the time.

I pack my stuff, shake hands all around, and exit into Saskatoon's windy snow.

Blessings come in various...

Blessings come in various shapes, as do warts. Insomnia, for example, as well as giving possible evidence of a troubled life, also allows extra time to observe the connections of the universe and occasionally even join an unscheduled partnership.

At 3:00 a.m. on this unusually warm, mid-winter night, a car approaches Kenora over the thin ice of Lake of the Woods. I watch from my lightless bedroom, hoping the car lights don't splash into deeper darkness. They don't, and I nod gratitude to the ice gods, then turn on my own lights and get up.

Friend Penny has taught me to grind the coffee beans just before the moment of brewing, and even though my buds can detect absolutely no difference in taste, I have come to depend on the ritual, especially at 3:00 a.m.

The beans get ground—Starbuck's Verona, as recommended by daughter Sarah—and I reach into my cupboard for a mug while the coffeemaker drips into the pot. Mid-reach, I stop the grasp as the stories of the mugs come at me from the shelf, competing and isolated histories, sad and happy, alive and gone. Why on this morning? On other days, I reach in and grab a mug, barely focusing on the handle let alone the history, and then move on. Today, the mugs jointly challenge me, in more and less (it varies) friendly fashion, forcing me to listen. The interweaving stories are these:

• My sister Sue gave me a huge, dark-green cup and saucer, which is occasionally used for long Saturday morning coffee and newspaper overdoses. I smile in her Peace River direction every time I use it;

• A white mug with red and black lettering sports my name and the crest of the New England Journal of Medicine. My usual lie, when visitors raise an eyebrow, is an aw-shucks admission to my recent appointment as Honorary Editor. The reality, of course, is that I paid $20 for it, answering a fund-raising offer in the Journal;

• An olive-brown, no-handle, glass-shaped mug is insulated on the bottom half and can be used for red wine or hot coffee, as has been proven by multiple testing episodes. It was bought at an artist's studio in Oyster Bed Bridge, Prince Edward Island, across the highway from the Cafe St Jean. It now has a chip from my carelessness;

• One of my favourite places to visit in northwestern Ontario is the WOODSHED, in Vermilion Bay. It sells gorgeous wood, ceramic and glass artistry, with an emphasis on the wooden, and is run by clever, friendly and skilled people. My beige mug, potbellied and thin-lipped, has four pine trees painted on two sides and is one of a set of three;

• A giant-sized, burgundy mug, holding about half a litre, was a gift from one of my daughters. I am fond of the colour burgundy;

• One of the mugs is rarely used. It is wide, shallow and thin, has a white background with a blue crest and words in Portuguese. It was a gift from a nurse friend in Black Tickle, Labrador, having been salvaged from a grounded fishing trawler in a windy harbour of the Island of Ponds. My friend died, but her memory is alive;

• A tall, heavy, white mug has a Ted Harrison painting on one side and was a gift from a lost friend in Dawson City, Yukon, following a shared sneak exit from a too-crowded conference in Whitehorse;

• There are three whale mugs on my shelf. One is black with a white patch, as with an Orca, and has a whale's tail for a handle. It is daughter Jan's, for when she visits. Another is a soft blue and has a raised humpback on the side; it was a gift from Ben, from the Winnipeg Folk Festival. I use it often; it is comfortable in my hand. The last option, with this same hand still poised in mid-air, is of a beige mug with many types of whale black-painted around the sides—minke, blue, sperm, humpback, and right—and was a gift from Ben, from our shared time on Grand Manan Island. It is a fog-study and walk-soaked memory holder.

<u>All</u> of the mugs are memory holders. The rush of images only lasts for a few seconds, until I pick a mug and pour the coffee. As I glance out the 3:15 a.m. window, the lake ice is moonlit, empty, and unbroken.

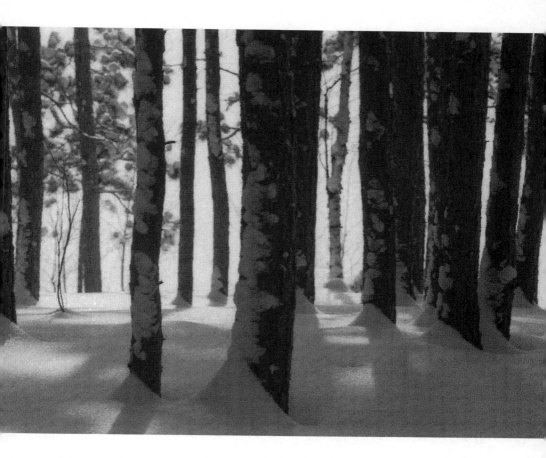

These are the trees of my childhood. The image signals the beginning of a great day tobogganing then warming up in the cabin with cocoa and chili. -BJ

From northern Canada...

*F*rom northern Canada, a friend who gathers images while listening to the sound of place writes:

"Things have settled down here. We had a difficult first week—problems with gear at first. It's antiquated and temperamental. We seemed to get about a half-day's work done each day. We are now up and running and on the right road.

I am sitting at my makeshift desk when Zach walks in, sees me, smiles, and comes over. 'How are you?' I say, and he says, 'A little better. I've been finding it really hard.' Later, I am sitting at the Take-Out, talking to the owner. He says, 'It was the hardest winter I ever went through. There were times when you were afraid for the phone to ring in case it was more bad news.'

And, then, one night, I was walking home. There was a building site on the way, the foundation of a new house. Inside was a bunch of kids that, at first, I took to be playing. What was really going on was two kids fighting in the middle and all the other kids hanging on the fringe, watching half-fascinated, half-terrified. One larger boy was choking a smaller one. I was about to intervene when another man shouted at him. He immediately let the young kid go, and the crisis was over. I knew the man, have known him for some time. I asked him how he was, how he was doing. He said he was doing well, although it had been a hard winter, a lot of deaths, a lot of suicides. Hard to help the families, he said. I asked again how he was doing himself. 'Pretty good. I just had two weeks off and spent all the time with the kids. It was real good.' That was the best thing I'd heard all week.

And, then, I met a friend from the old days. She said, 'You've changed. You used to be different—so nice and open and honest. Now you're different, more guarded or something, not as nice.' My fear, of course, is that it could be true. She also said she thought it was because I was spending too much time in the south. She said, 'You belong here.' I think I fear that might be true as well. But it's the land I love—even more than the people.

Even in town I am touched by the landscape and the skies. I was walking back home the other night and I saw the Big Dipper hanging over the hill, wreathed by aurora. If you had asked me where the Big Dipper was, I wouldn't have been able to tell you, but seeing it in that place was so familiar to me. I knew it fit and that I'd seen it right there in that same place a dozen times before. I regret being tied to the edit room and not being able to get out of town. Jump aboard a boat and head off around the corner. North and south; it wouldn't matter.

That's all for now. I might get another note off before I leave here at the end of the week."

Migration is a multifaceted...

Migration is a multifaceted phenomenon involving varying needs for warmth and sustenance, mobility for mobility's sake, random searching for a different colour of light on open air, inherited group behaviour, and a not-so-simple personal need for a change in stimuli. It appears, when one lives on the edge of Lake of the Woods, that migration is a seagull's breakfast.

Both the gulls and some humans take a seasonal opportunity to scram for a while, usually going south or west, and then we return. When I come back after a week away, tired and rejuvenated from walking, writing and hiding from contact, I drive into Kenora, at 7:00 p.m., in mid-April. The stretch of road running along to the railroad overpass, less than a kilometre from the huge statue of a muskie at the west side of the town harbour, is one of my favourite visual treats in Canada. The harbour, waterfront buildings and nearby islands, as well as the water's edge sidewalk and the railroad tracks built into the side of the steep hill, all combine to give a harmonious sweep. This view at dusk is spectacular, with a characteristic enveloping purple light seeping into all lines of sight, along with the land's contrasting shades of colour and tone, and the buildings' lights standing out as a foil.

In late spring, all summer, and in early fall, I give myself as many chances as I can to take this walk soon after sundown. The type of beautiful urban vista I'm describing isn't something you can fake; it's either there to be blended into or it isn't, and the key lies in the blending. My favourites, and I'm talking about views not places, include Banff's main street, with Cascade Mountain as a backdrop; West Van and downtown Vancouver, as seen from the seawall at Stanley Park; the view of old St. John's from the Battery; downtown Toronto from the Island; and this short stretch of Kenora. While the aptly maligned planner types can't fake it, they certainly can wreck it, and it could be argued that they and we specialize in that tendency. Kenora has done some of the right things along some of its waterfront, eventually and partially and especially when viewed at dusk.

On this day there is also a once-a-year bonus, as the seagulls have returned while I was gone. They are everywhere, hundreds of them, sitting on the frozen harbour as scattered patches of white on darkening ice, flying in thick flocks over the railroad tracks and circling as a huge group over the town's mall and grocery stores, taking loud, wide spirals over the widening patches of open water, and everywhere crying their song. They flock when they return, much more so than for the rest of the spring and summer, and I have to remember to find the reason, to ask or read or preferably to intuit.

I grew up in Nova Scotia where the gulls never leave and so don't congregate in this dramatic, large-crowd, opening-day fashion. I'm reminded of the surprised awe I felt on seeing the migration of geese for the first time, in Manitoba. During a Maritime childhood, far from the geese's flight paths, I'd seen pictures and read of the geese's V-patterns and high-up audible calls and so recognized the event but was still incredulous.

The seagulls' return to Lake of the Woods is different, with a less-heralded group randomness. Improvisational drama is a personal favourite, and I try to keep the glee to myself as I watch the gulls settle in for the summer. It is fine to see them again, and I don't want to risk spoiling it. There is always a possibility that they could become scared or annoyed, leading to an unplanned migration, a spontaneous search for greyer ice. The sound of their cries at 5:00 a.m. on an April morning is welcome reward for this cautious pessimism.

The gulls are not so inhibited as they fly in their spring flocks, scream with ambiguous vigour, and are generally full of airborne fuss. They are back.

Laura Smith is a singer...

L aura Smith is a singer-songwriter, a Canadian who has been mobile from coast to artistically impecunious coast, and many of us haven't heard sung words from her in years. Observation of Canadian artists has taught me that creativity is a difficult way to feed oneself, if you insist on the necessity of food. Building visions from mental ashes is often personally entertaining and occasionally culturally enlightening, but don't count on financial viability and definitely don't bet the farm, not even the farm.

This perception of a country that is artistically rich but insists on most artists being poor arises from lifelong peering about as well as episodic eye-to-eye contact with dancers, painters, writers, photographers, actors, musicians, and a scattered singer-songwriter.

Laura Smith, to circle back to the specific, weaves moving and insightful lyrics with intricate and cohesive melodies, and she has been writing and sharing these songs from both coasts. She is capable of celebrating and lamenting without alleging the inevitability of either. Her connections are emotionally profound and often flirt with a loss of control or of bothering with control. She is a wonderfully-frightening presence, and it seems that most Canadians have never heard her.

One of Laura Smith's songs, "Armistice Day," is linked to Vancouver's *Sylvia Hotel*. She uses images of this aging, room-renting, waterside, vine-covered matriarch to reflect our ability to draw from the sea and our longing for a lasting armistice. She recognizes the connections. It's a brilliantly evocative and hopeful hymn to tides and time, a signpost for whenever we find ourselves grounded anywhere near our own False Creek.

While again staying at the *Sylvia*, so that I may connect words while sitting at a small desk near a window in room 325, alternating with walks along the rain-soaked seawall, I notice how often the various inner wanderings come back to Laura Smith, to her words: *"I am in a hotel that hung banners on Armistice Day. I hold up well beside the water; I was made that way."*

Later in the week, as I'm retrieving my room key after twelve kilometres on the seawall and Denman Avenue, a quiet-lobby moment occurs involving only me and the front-desk person. I ask if they have enjoyed being celebrated by Laura Smith, by her song. Which song, I'm asked, and who is Laura Smith? I explain in about three sentences and then offer to send a tape, no charge, "all part of the service," suggesting that their quality of life will take a leap forward, if that can be imagined, gesturing at the rain-lashed windows and empty lobby. The offer is met with cool disinterest.

As I attempt to capture this memory-ghost, at 6:30 a.m. in the gradually-opening, underground food court of Montreal's Centre-Ville complex, while nursing a large, strong coffee, there is background music tempering the clatter and sulky fatigue of shops being opened and workaholics nosily striding the aisles toward offices. The music is wonderfully evocative, controlled and almost edgy but without adrenalin or challenge, and while I have no idea of the source, I lift my paper cup to salute the classy Quebecois; no one notices, and the music continues.

A half-hour later, as I leave the food-shop section and enter the wide, tiled echo chamber underground tunnel system leading to the Palais des Congres de Montreal, the source of the music becomes evident. A middle-aged man is standing mid tunnel playing a saxophone with a small music-making machine by his feet, as is a sax case, open for money. I slow to deposit coins, we nod at each other, and I continue walking.

4:30 a.m., at Dawson Creek...

4:30 a.m., at Dawson Creek, northern BC—This is a fine time of night to wake, as the hotel is quiet and the air in the room is cool; it is just the right time. The curtains have been left partly open, as always, on the premise that some light will accommodate sleep vision better than darkness ever can. Rolling over to the left side will sometimes lead back to sleep but usually does not.

7:30 a.m., Flight #1691 departs Dawson Creek for Vancouver— The plane is a Beechcraft 1900D, a twin-engine eighteen-seater with eleven people seated and two of these are pilots. There is no washroom. Off the left wing are mountains back-dropped by a sunrise. It is beautiful, all of it, and I let it shine on my face, through the window. There is new snow on the tops and upper sides of the mountains, with evergreen trees carpeting further down the slopes and in the valleys. There are high lakes in hanging valleys and scattered rain ponds, and none are frozen, not yet. There are also rivers twisting around, always finding the low route. We are cruising at 525 km/hr and at 24,000 non-metric feet, eagerly avoiding all low routes, for a while.

9:30 a.m., landing at Vancouver—We have approached Vancouver by coming in over the coastal mountains, the lower Sunshine Coast, Bowen Island, and then in low over the water just off Stanley Park and the entrance to False Creek, finally coasting over the flatland of Delta and the runways. As I leave the plane and find the gate for the flight to Calgary, there are mountains to be seen from the airport windows, ordinary airport windows with sharp-edged mountains just over there; amazing, every time. There is sun, grass and leaves, all of these flowing every which way, gentle bright on green on framing height. I'm in love, yet again. (Vancouver ignores me, yet again.) The plane leaves for Calgary, with me in place.

Noon, Calgary—The flight from Vancouver gets into Calgary twelve minutes before my flight to Saskatoon is to leave. We have angled in over Banff, more or less, so I am already wistful about the shared times in Calgary and Banff with daughter-J. As I hustle toward the semi-distant gate, the Air Canada minions are lined up along the halls and aisles, shouting at me to snap out of this incipient funk, making side bets and cheering me on as the clock ticks toward departure time, whacking my butt with stale flight food whenever I slow down and generally being their usual jolly and helpful selves. (I make the flight.)

3:00 p.m., Saskatoon—In the baggage area, I find that my bag also made the flight, and I mentally apologize to The People's Airline. In the parking lot, I find that my car's tires are still inflated and the motor starts; life is forgiving. I get lost for thirty minutes getting out of the city, just to balance things. I'm trying to find the Yellowhead route to Yorkton and on to Manitoba and Kenora, and a citizen in a Seven/ Eleven store comes to my rescue, giving clear and helpful directions. I thank him, with full eye contact, and ask if he wants a free ride to Kenora, one-way. He declines, with a smile.

7:00 p.m., east of Yorkton—After only forty-five minutes of searching, the World Series game is found on Saskatchewan rural radio, clear, perfect reception, and I do a seated version of the wave. The sun has gone down somewhere behind me, probably near Vancouver, and traffic is light, so I get the car on cruise, turn off the dash lights, and cheer on the new team of the new millennium—the Arizona Diamondbacks for pity's sake—as they beat up on the team of the past millennium—the New York Yankees. New York, the city that is, could stand a victory or two this fall, and I admit that I would not grieve to see them win it, but the baseball gods work in deeply weird ways. Using my cell phone, I call the aptly self-labeled Baseball Babe in Winnipeg and we compare impressions of the game from the different angles of TV watcher and radio listener. Our impressions coincide.

10:30 p.m., Portage la Prairie, Manitoba—I'm starting to get sleepy, seeing deer where there aren't any, not yet blinking hard or weaving about, but I'm thinking about it so it's time to stop, and only three hours from home. I pull into a motel, startling the desk clerk, as there are only four cars in the acres of parking lot. When I'm in my room, I call Ben and attempt to fake her into thinking she had bet $20 on the Yankees. The attempt fails. In fact, it appears that I owe her $10, but I'm suspicious of how this played out.

9:30 a.m., Kenora—The car finds its way into my parking slot at the Health Unit, and it is fine to be home. It is always a relief to feel that way.

A travelling dancer writes from...

Atravelling dancer writes from a cybercafe in Europe:

"I am in Berlin, the city after Manhattan is taken.

Last night I took a night train from Warsaw to Berlin. The train was an hour late, so we didn't leave Warsaw until after midnight, and I didn't sleep right away, probably not until around 2:00 a.m. It was supposed to get in at 7:00 a.m., but I thought that being an hour late leaving and all that we'd get in an hour late; does that not make sense? So, I am sleepy sleeperson and the conductor guy knocks on my door at 6:45 a.m. or something and asks if I want coffee. I said, 'no, thanks,' but what I thought was, 'Why are you disturbing my slumber?' Looking back on the situation, I guess I was supposed to get up at this time. So, I go back to sleep and get up around 20 minutes later. When I go out to the washroom in bare feet and sweats, a whole lot of business people are standing waiting to get off the train and looked at me kind of amused. I was like, *'whatever,'* and go pee, and then go back to my room. I then decide that I want to know where we are, and I look out my little window and AHHHH!!! WE ARE IN BERLIN! Who knew?

I have never piled 4 bags on myself so quickly.

I went straight to the airport and tried to change my ticket with Lufthansa ('The German Airline'): 'No, we cannot change your ticket; you have to go to this travel agent; it is twenty minutes away; they open at 9:00 a.m.; maybe you can get on a flight today though.' I store my luggage, after swearing for 10 minutes at my freakin trolley thing that desperately wants to turn left through the crowded Berlin airport. 'No,' I plead. 'Go straight!' but it is persistent. I take a cab to the travel agent address, and it doesn't open until 10:00 a.m., so I slope around. Then it opens, and there is no flight until Friday—4 days.

I am distressed. I want to go home. But then the wonderful travel agent looks up other flights, and *I booked one for tomorrow*, to London, then Toronto. And I get 40% of money back, so I think I actually get a *better* deal! **Hurrah!**

I leave Berlin tomorrow at 7ish, and I am just going to stay at the airport tonight. People will definitely stay away.

So, all that is left is negotiating from Toronto to Winnipeg.

I can't wait to see you."

Sarah and I have been book wandering...

Sarah and I have been book wandering at Indigo, near Bay and Bloor, Toronto. Book wandering is different from book shopping, as it involves letting the tides of whim and aisle, crowd and sight and reflex, just guide you along, drift you.

We have both been relieved to find out that neither took offense to the other's inclination to book wander alone, meeting every so often to compare finds and searches and to connect before going off separately again, alone and linked. (Books will link you while alone.)

My home in Kenora has hundreds of these linkages, these lifelines, in bookcases and on tables around most of the rooms, and occasionally piled on floors, open and closed, partially read or lying in wait. Many of these will never be read, and that is not a problem. They are magic under cover, just as potent and awesome when closed, perhaps never to be opened. It takes courage and recklessness to open them without knowing the consequences.

Sarah and I have ambled around for over an hour, and we have to go; we're tired, and we both have promises to keep. We pay our bills and start out the Bay Street door. Ahead of us are two people, a woman and a man, both in their mid to late twenties. They are talking and carrying bags of books. He goes out the door, and she follows, and I reflexly prepare to catch the heavy door swinging back at me, carelessly unheld, the way city people so often do it, civility being crushed by the weight of numbers. The woman defeats my bias with nonchalant ease, a simple warm gesture of her day. She not only holds the door for me, but she also looks me full in the eyes and smiles an acknowledgement to my "thank you" and then does the same for Sarah. The man doesn't seem pleased, with an oh-for-God's-sake-let's-*go* look on his cool face.

Sarah and I watch them walk on ahead, and then we talk of the moment, of the woman's eyes and smile, her casual and useful warmth, and of our hope that she finds more rewarding companions. We were already close, a daughter and a father who love each other and continue to build connections and shared values, and this city person just gave us an additional gift, a bonus <u>and</u> an antidote.

Bay Street feels friendly and supportive as we stroll home on this damp February evening. Having met a role model, I make plans to be a better city person, when I visit.

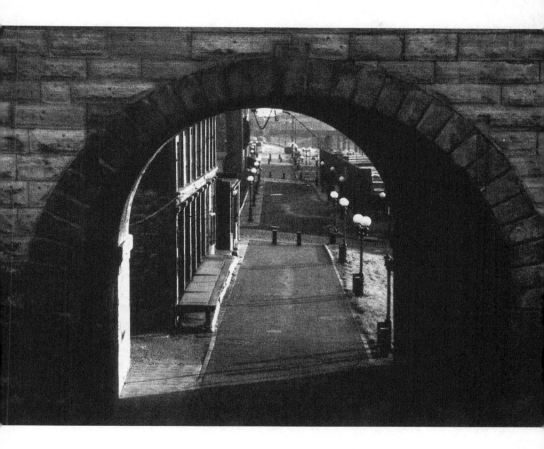

Waterfront revitalization but no one walked the promenades, sat on the benches or ventured to stroll the Mississippi at St. Louis. -BJ

On the wall of a person who is overdue...

*O*n the wall of a person who is overdue to be on the positive rolling end of a wave of good luck is a picture of a mother and daughter, ages then about 35 and 15. Both are cut from the same cocky, look-you-in-the-eye-and-laugh mould, side by side, related and different.

I think of this aging scene as I watch the daughter from the picture, now herself a mother with her own 5-year-old daughter, in the Market Garden Cafeteria of the Delta Chelsea Hotel, in Toronto, just off Yonge St., near Ryerson University. I let them go on ahead, so I just watch their movements and the subsequent reactions of the tray-piling and table-sitting diners.

These are two visual magnets, with startling facial features and wild hair, long skirts and rough sweaters, and a completely nonchalant disregard for their stand-out style. The five-year-old is relaxed in the midst of the busy, confused, stop-and-go flow of the tired, hungry, come-from-away, noon-hour, adult cafeteria crowd. The big people notice her, but she doesn't notice them. This is definitely *not* a stereotypic cute-kid, showing off in the land of the giants; this is simply a confident, smart, independent person. I remember her mother at the same age, and her grandmother at age 15, and am again intrigued by the depth of influence exerted by genes when combined with teaching by example.

The other diners are also intrigued, with heads turning and many with appreciative or puzzled expressions. The Chelsea attracts a middle-class business and sports crowd, and they are not used to aliens in their midst; everybody's cool, no offense given or taken.

I take their picture, mother and daughter, in my mind, for my own wall.

At Deck 27 of the Delta Chelsea Hotel...

*A*t Deck 27 of the Delta Chelsea Hotel in Toronto—the "Adult Fitness Centre" (kids have to go to their own pool on the second floor)—there are treadmills that face huge windows, allowing the sweaty walkers and joggers to look directly across to an apartment building. This view may be boring or fascinating, depending on one's attitude. (Is there any truer truism than the ". . . in the eye of the beholder..." recognition? You may try to tell me there is one, but I don't think I'll let myself see it.)

I'm in this hotel on a Saturday morning because of Friday and Monday meetings bracketed around the weekend. Even if there were no upcoming earth-saving, conclusion-guaranteed, intelligence-soaked session for Monday, I'd *still* be here on a Saturday, because the airfares are about a thousand dollars cheaper, Winnipeg-Toronto return, if you stay over the Saturday night, and you can't cancel or change for any reason. The time-of-my-weekend-life versus taxpayers' money—no contest; I lose.

No problem; I get to see my daughter, step-mother, brother, sister, brother-in-law, and nieces, my family, and thanks from me to the generous taxpayers, including (I must add) to myself. I'm musing like this, about the vagaries of taxation justice, as I plod along the treadmill's highway on the 27th floor. Across the way is the apartment building of angles and windows, all modern and crisp in shades of adobe, salmon, beige, and washed-out green. It is close to us, only about the width of a narrow street away. We are both cliff dwellers, those adobe clean-cut types and us sweaty plodders, separated by a narrow space. We both live near the top of the canyon walls, (which is only a good thing if you're fond of long falls), and we don't interact, not even to exchange shouts. We do, however, peer into each other's bedrooms and treadmill centres, a connection of sorts.

As I look across, I notice several things about the other side. They have very few plants in their windows, and one or two still have strings of lights hanging on from some festival of glitter. My line of view includes eight stories, the top eight, and so about 32 apartments. I peer at and into windows, hoping for a glimpse of something completely different, a spark of originality and (dare I hope it?) defiance amidst this jungle of cool beige. Finally I spot it, the subversive loner, the standard-bearer for non-conformity, the red sheep, nonchalant and carefree in the midst of the wolves. (Why keep one's biases buried? What's the gain?) I've noticed that almost all the apartments have those stiff vertical blinds on the windows, with a couple of old-fashioned horizontal tin types as well. There *is* one, just one of the thirty-two, that has fabric drapes, gathered at their waist, hanging in a way that allows for folds and curves.

I complete my 2.4 miles on the treadmill, (which is resolutely American in its resistance to metric distance), and nod a salute to the person or persons who resist the neo-hard and straight, and instead dare to drape themselves in soft. There is no reply, across the gap.

Fourteen of us are in a high-ceilinged...

Fourteen of us are in a high-ceilinged boardroom on the 15th floor of an old stone building on a central avenue in Toronto. The large double doors to the room have golden borders and handles, and they are framed by marble columns to the sides and a marble slab high to the top. The rectangular table is long and heavy looking with its thick mahogany-coloured surface, and it's surrounded by padded swivel chairs that have arms. The walls have a dark-beige textured paneling, with pictures of six older men scattered along one wall. These pictures are placed without any discernable sense of order, style or humour; these are our culture's equivalent of dogs marking the borders of their territory. I make a mental vow to stay zipped.

There are flip charts, an overhead projector with screen pulled down, and a slide projector on a lectern in the corner, all of these ready to go should serious discussion break out. This room has many relatives scattered across Canada, such as A106 at the University of Manitoba's medical school. My take on such spaces is that, unless you are yourself an oppressor, the room is oppressive. If I feel any level of comfort and familiarity inside this stuffy, elitist, humourless, sexist, and antiquated display of power, I'm going to keep it to myself.

On this day we are an evidence-based group, more or less, thick with degrees and titles, most of us. There is numerical gender equity, a pair of sevens. Three or four wear wedding rings, with one indulging in relaxed ambiguity or rebellion as the band is on the "wrong" finger. One woman stands with her back to the door's marble edge, and I assume that we all make a mental diagnosis of low-back pain. Four of the seven men wear ties, and none of the fourteen people wear glasses. Only one is left-handed, confirming my hunch that we are a non-sinister group.

One woman knits, episodically. As I watch her, and this is only the second meeting we've shared, it seems that she uses the knitting as a self-control device, bringing it out when she wants to force herself to just observe, to sit on the periphery for a while, listening, gathering pearls. I like this person, her face and the content and style of what she says, and most of all for what it seems that she's working for. She used to be an American and has retained the in-your-face confidence, not exhibiting the stereotypic Canadian reluctance to stand out by challenging the average. When she knits, she becomes much more Canadian. I prefer the atmosphere and the results when her needles are on the table and her eyes and voice are roaming, but my mother was born in the U.S., so my chromosomes and reflexes are suspect. Come to think of it, I was born in Toronto, so both my nature *and* my nurture are in full trouble.

As I watch the room, I'm struck by the extent of my ambivalence. I'd like to interact less often with such rooms and more often with such knitters. However, it is becoming more and more evident that my range of influence regarding the flow of my own life is extremely limited. In spite of this, the urge to battle the current of the day, or to even attempt to change the course of the stream, continues to surface. When the knitter packs up her stuff, having to leave early, and nods to the room as she departs, I just smile and nod back. The encounter will remain sufficient unto itself. Reality is such an unforgiving parent to the moment.

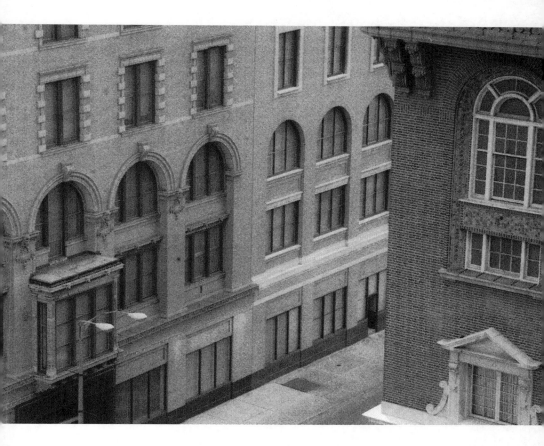

Great windows but no light gets in; what's the story? -BJ

There are three ferry docks...

T here are three ferry docks on Toronto Island, all a five-to ten-minute sail from the downtown. One is at Ward's Island, at the east end of the connected mid-city-harbour sandbar archipelago. This area is where people live, and the dock is open all year, which the residents probably appreciate. Another is on Centre Island and it's the tourist focus, therefore only open during the warmer months when tourists dare to mingle and peer. The other one is at Hanlan's Point, at the west end of the five-kilometre-long skinny group of islands, smack beside the island airport. There are buoys extending out from the airstrip into the natural straight-line path of the ferry, causing it to circle slightly as it approaches and leaves Hanlan's Point. The buoys are part of the landing and take-off pathway, and occasionally a small plane will come in low over the ferry—a nice touch, so long as it doesn't.

Hanlan's is the least used dock of the three, although those aiming for the nearby nude beach and most summer bicyclists usually take this one, as do some of the patrons and staff of the nearby Gibraltar Point

Centre for the Arts. Any car or truck going to the Island has to use this ferry, such as the Thursday grocery delivery and the weekday school bus. In spite of all this, it is the least used and runs less frequently than the others, or that's how it feels when you stay at Gibraltar Point. It's definitely a less crowded run, quieter for walking to and from and for riding on the much smaller boat. Some of us gravitate that way. It is, however, a lonely dark walk at night, if you've come in on the day's last run in late September. As you walk, you hope this is not your unlucky night.

Hanlan's Point is named after Ned Hanlan, who lived on the island. He was born in 1855 and died in 1908, was 5 ft. 9 in. tall and weighed 150 pounds, and he was a superb oarsman. In 1880 and again in 1884, he was the world champion in single sculls. There is an evocative mural of Hanlan, complete with historical details, on the wall of the Rectory Café on Ward Island. In the portrayal he appears to be fit and determined.

From the benches near Ned's dock, there's a mixed urban and marine panorama, night or day, when you are facing north, facing the city. The city offers its best face from this distance, better by far than up close and also better than from an airplane arriving or even leaving. Many of the advertising celebrations of Toronto are taken from the Island—a few trees, a safe expanse of water, and then there's the city, framed to be grand. Toronto is inviting and benevolent, from this angle.

Occasionally, I have sat on these benches, waiting for the ferry to take me across to watch the Blue Jays play ball. From the bench it's a direct-line look to the Skydome, usually dome-closed but maybe open in the late afternoon before the night game, if the weather is good and if they have remembered to flip the switch.

Near these benches and the ferry dock is a small black boulder, about three-quarters of a metre high and wide, which has a slightly smaller plaque mounted on it. The boulder is just off the road, near a tree—no fanfare, no big deal. The text on the weathered plaque reads:

> **Near this site, at the old Hanlan's Point Stadium, on 5 Sept 1914, baseball's legendary Babe Ruth hit his first home run as a professional—the only home run he ever hit in the minor leagues. The lanky 19-year-old rookie, playing for the Providence Greys in the International League, connected with a pitch off Ellis Johnson of the Toronto Maple Leafs, sending the ball over the fence in right field and scoring three runs for his team. Ruth, as pitcher of his team, allowed only one hit and the Greys shut out Toronto 9—0. His later career made Babe Ruth a monumental figure in baseball history.**
>
> **This plaque commemorates both the extraordinary career of Babe Ruth and the important contribution made by Toronto to the game of baseball from "little league" teams to the Toronto Blue Jays of the American League. (1985)**

The ferry arrives, loads a few foot passengers and one van and leaves for the city terminal, angling a semi-circle past the airport's landing buoys. We don't cheat and cut across, but it must be tempting because there's no plane in sight and it seems as if we can see a long way.

A walk to the ballpark...

A walk to the ballpark in Toronto, in almost warm late-afternoon April sun, is a twenty-minute striding stroll from the Delta Chelsea at Gerrard and Yonge, criss-crossing down and over, over and down, west toward the CN Tower and south toward the lake, finally settling for a casual pace along the east side of University Avenue. This is an episodically wonderful street, wide as a European boulevard with a series of parks in the middle which permit sitting and watching, purposeful urban hesitation. It's empty in April, with no one sleeping on the benches or sitting on the steps of the monuments, and the cars passing on either side feel close, immediate. Later in summer there will be the baffling shade of trees and the full sound of flowers overriding the traffic. Today, I keep moving.

There is a moment in the walk when I realize I'm in the midst of my own adventure, a partially earned gift to be savoured and protected, and possibly shared. Such flashes of connected elation are, it has become apparent, easily lost in the grasping and also tragically easy to harm in others, especially in ones loved. I think about this along the wide sidewalk of University Avenue. The scanning happiness and sense of warm possibility nevertheless persist; on some days the gift is well-wrapped.

As I amble, less striding now, crossing Dundas and then Queen, past Richmond and Adelaide, moving toward the looping veer of the bottom of University, before it changes direction and does a reverse metamorphosis from swan to the ugly duckling of Yonge, I get ready to cross the wide street, thinking about jaywalking for a flickering, suicidal moment before rejecting that option and aiming instead for the crowded and conformist crosswalk at the next intersection.

Just ahead of me, midway between King and Wellington, a man comes out of a coffee place, holding a large, lidded, take-out cardboard cup as if it's precious. He is wearing semi-conservative office clothes, shirt and tie, with no jacket, good pants and shoes, and the socks match, at a glance. (My workplace clothes-conscious critics would be proud of this guy, possibly offering a "*See?*" of directive advice.) He is moving slowly and looking around, going back to an acceptable job with a medicinal coffee for the early evening. He doesn't hesitate, not a beat missed, as he steps into the rush-hour traffic, calmly weaves to the mid-street illusionary island of painted *don't-go-here* stripes, then drifts into more between-car weaving to the opposite sidewalk, four lanes of obstacle-thick negotiation, one hand in a pocket and the other cradling a cup. He is not posing casual but is the real thing, having done this many times before. He's at home.

I stop to watch. As I'm behind him on the sidewalk, he has no idea that he is providing entertainment or direction. I consider following his lead and his style but then shake my head and continue walking toward the crosswalk, recognizing that I'd be dead or arrested within ten seconds out there in this foreign world's homicidal traffic. It is necessary to pick one's spots.

At Front Street the light lets me cross without pausing, on cue, flashing a permissive smile, acknowledging the shared cadence and humour of the city.

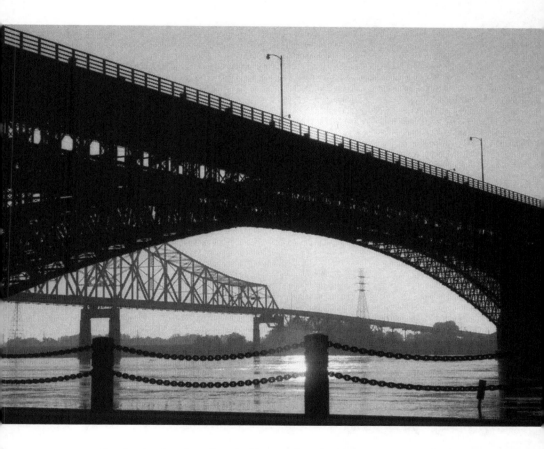

Bridge built when baseball was played only on grass. -BJ

A few times in one recent summer...

A few times in one recent summer, to give a sharp example of how our roads unwind in strange and personal ways, I was driving with the radio and tape player both turned off and the sunroof open, moving at about 100 km/hr, when I heard the entire clear loud song of a field bird. I can't understand how it could happen, not at that speed and with all the wind-rush sound, but it *was* there, the whole call, lasting for two to three seconds. Perhaps the bird was fast-flying in the same direction I was driving and calling as it flew? Or I imagined the end of the call, a blood memory? It doesn't matter; I heard it. I was alone and driving, clear-eyed, awake, and visited by song, once again privileged to be allowed to be there.

In the winter that followed, on the slowly unwinding road between Fort Frances and Kenora, there was another quick burst of sight, a view permitted past my own edge. Off to the side of the road, near Nestor Falls, were three large moose, not moving, just watching or waiting for me to pass so they could cross my narrow, short-sighted, noisy and

glimpse – Pete Sarsfield

dangerous flat path and get back into their clear, dark home woods. I remember someone saying, "when you're lost, take the path," but these moose knew better.

One of the joys of having cable TV...

*O*ne of the joys of having cable TV, ranking well ahead of being able to choose from a wide variety of skilled portrayals of death and despair, is the opportunity to have multiple baseball games available, from April to October. (November to March is just a 7th inning stretch, a pitching change, a rain delay; it'll go by quickly, and then we'll get back to the game.) As I'm making supper, cleaning up, doing laundry, answering mail, all the usual and necessary mundanities, I can choose from the Blue Jays, Cubs, Dodgers, Braves, White Sox, and on a rare good-fortune day, the close-to-my-heart Expos. I find that the sound of the game, even coming unwatched from the other room, eases the day along. It is a background chant, and it soothes. I'm a baseball fan.

On this hot summer evening in Kenora, I've got a breeze coming in through all my windows off the Lake of the Woods, easing the 30°C humidity. I'm putting groceries away, still trying to find the best fit for things after two years in my apartment, and on one bag-laden kitchen trek, I pause at the door to the living room, to glance at the game.

The hitter fouls one into the stands, a soft looping fly ball well down the first baseline. The camera picks up a fan with a glove making a routine catch, and then zooms in on him standing there with his arms elevated in the classic victory pose, the final game of the World Series having been rescued by this spectacular grab. The camera doesn't hang in there, but at a glance it does *not* appear that the fans around the foul-catcher are rising to their feet in a standing O.

On the next pitch there's a vicious line shot, foul again, this time into the stands right behind third base. The camera person is now into this and quickly focuses on the flight of the ball. We see it ricochet off several outstretched hands before it slows, and a man reaches for it, in the air just off to his side, both hands, no glove. He fumbles it, hands of stone, and the ball flicks back another couple of rows. Beside the man is a boy of about seven or eight, and he looks up at the man, surprised, incredulous. The man looks straight ahead. The camera goes back to the game.

On the road between Thunder Bay and Kenora...

O n the road between Thunder Bay and Kenora, near Ignace, a BLUE RODEO song is played on the radio. It helps me remember the recent winter evening this band came to Muskrat Dam and were respectful.

For most of my adult life, I've witnessed entertainers visit northern communities and be disrespectful, not always but often. This happened in places as dissimilar and widely spaced as Norway House, Cambridge Bay, Nain, Cartwright, and Northwest River and was usually characterized by either a condescending attitude or a bored and underachieving dismissal. My guess is that sometimes this response comes from simple alien fear because of their overwhelming unfamiliarity with the region and its people. We never *ever* want to let the audience see us sweat, do we?

BLUE RODEO was *glad* to be there, in the middle of the winter, with kids running around and only a few hundred people in the auditorium. The police at the margins were completely unnecessary as peace keepers, so they just watched and laughed and became part of the spectators. The band also seemed to join its own audience, without self-congratulation or fuss, as they displayed their connection by tone of voice, as well as the words spoken, and by the intensity of their music. We were important to them, and they dared to make themselves vulnerable by letting this show. As a result, they became even more important to us.

There was a moment of cross-cultural misunderstanding at the end of the set, and it was both revealing and touching. The band finished, thanked the audience for a wonderful evening, and left the stage, just putting the instruments down by the amps. In their culture, that of southern and musical Canada, if the audience claps and cheers enthusiastically, the performers will come back for an *aw-shucks-if-you-insist* encore. It's a ritual, and we're used to it, or some of us are. Most of the people in the auditorium at Muskrat Dam, however, assumed that, if you say *thanks folks, I'm done*, then you <u>are</u> done and it would be rude to argue with your decision. A few ritualistic southern types stood up and indicated by words and actions that, if we clap, they'll come back and they'll be glad to do it. So we did, most of us did, and the band returned, perhaps a bit sheepishly or confused, but I have been known to project these emotions. The encore was warm and lengthy, a skilled, vibrant and shared respectfulness.

Near Ignace, I turn up the radio and keep driving.

From the summer train...

From the summer train between Truro, Nova Scotia, and Moncton, New Brunswick, a friend writes:

"I'm on the train. We have just shunted back and forth, and they announced the departure, yet we have been here for twenty minutes.

We're rolling out of the station, slowly passing the houses in the sun. An old couple sits outside an apartment building, warming memories as the train passes by. The whistle blows, and the train speeds up. I love the Tantramar marshland—muddy streams twisting through it. Seagulls fly away; ducks swim in the shallow ponds; wet mudbanks of the river reflect the overcast sky, a purple hue—my favourite colour.

The sun shines with warmth through the window. A portable CD player is blasting the ears of the fellow in the seat ahead of me. Shall I tell him that he'll be deaf before he's 50? A baby cries. The older couple across the aisle worry that the baby will whine all the way...they mutter to themselves.

We just went through a railroad crossing. I stared at the cars as they waited for the train to pass. I try to imagine where they are going. Do they, as when I am them, try to imagine what the blond-haired woman (peering over her reading glasses) is doing, where she is going?

The older woman across the aisle asks drowsily, 'Where are we now?' We've just passed Dorchester Penitentiary. I once spent a week there—well, not actually a week in Dorchester. I chose it for my Community Health experience while in nursing school at St. Martha's in Antigonish.

Well, Pete, my friend, it has been a good trip."

My daughter Sarah once said...

My daughter Sarah once said to me, "You make up memories." She didn't seem to mind; the memories fit.

CBC radio creates memories, and they fit. Late on a Saturday evening, a friend calls to say, "Turn on your radio. Dutchie Mason is playing." I do that and then sit in my lights-out living room with Dutch's aging voice embellishing our blues, including CBC's. A few days later, another friend email-writes, "Can you tap out a quick version of your story about the time you and Dutchie Mason were waiting tables...? I want to use it to support a request...I have my memory of the story, but I want to make sure that I get it right."

About forty years ago, Dutchie and I both served tables at the Cornwallis Inn, in Kentville, Nova Scotia, but that was almost all we had in common. His skill as a waiter and his history of being a musician who had played guitar for Jerry Lee Lewis, along with his intimidating street smarts and married status and the sidebar fact that the old hotel's domineering maitre d' was his mother, combined to put us in different realities. He spoke to me when our weaving paths crossed, but it was as a man might speak to a child. I decided, as I served the soup, that his tone indicated I was potentially a worthy child.

The large, brick hotel would receive bus tours all summer, with older Americans intent on experiencing the naive rural charms of the Annapolis Valley. One deliciously warm Sunday morning, when any sane person should have been outside playing ball or in bed sleeping off a hangover, Dutch and I were both serving breakfast in the subdued, high-ceilinged dining room. I wanted to be at the ballpark, and he wanted to be sleeping.

My waiter's attentiveness quotient was suffering as I focused on the free-theatre performance unfolding at Dutch's nearby table. Four tourists could not decide on orange juice versus apple, nor on bran flakes versus oatmeal, tea or coffee, milk or cream. They were in a quandary but didn't realize the extent; Dutchie was going to blow. I said to my table, also adrift on the sea of indecision, "Would you mind holding that thought, for *just* a minute? I'd like to watch this."

Dutch was wearing, as was I, the hotel's pretentious monkey suit for waiters, with fitted jacket, bow tie, cummerbund, and black pants. His one dress-code violation, always, involved footwear; he wore sandals, no socks. His maitre d' mother looked the other way but only for him. One of his sandaled feet began to tap, and he said, "Ladies, will you excuse me? I may be back," and he walked out of the dining room. I followed, from a safe distance. Dutch strode into the empty ballroom, went to the far end where a piano was perched in lonely splendour on a small, low stage, sat himself on the bench, adjusted some piano things, and then ripped out a full and loud version of Jerry Lee's "*Great Balls of Fire*." I stood at the back as the large room echoed and the waves spread to the sleepy town, the empty ballpark and the comfortable valley. I should have applauded but didn't, being fearful and perhaps a bit street smart myself. He then walked past me, without speaking or glancing, and went back to the dining room. "Now, ladies, was that apple or orange?" he asked.

A few years later, when I was overwhelmingly lonely in Halifax, I went to see him play a hotel lounge in Dartmouth, just across the bridge. His star was rising, but there were very few people in the lounge and even those were drinking and talking, not listening. By this time, I had a beard and long hair, still didn't wear sandals, and my star continued to be remarkably self-contained. He didn't know me from any other semi-drunk stranger in an uncaring, slack-assed, dead-end bar.

Dutch was remarkable, playing with intensity, skill and integrity, playing for the music. I sat well back, all the easier to watch, and after each of his numbers, I clapped full and loud. Dutch looked across at me, every time, pointed in my direction and said, "*You*, sir, are more than fair."

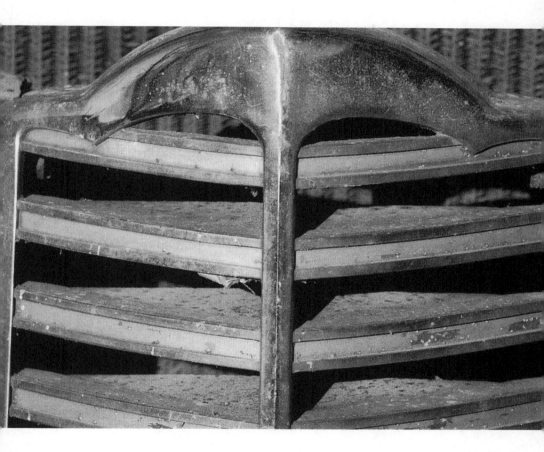

This grill belongs to a 1940-something that had an eight cylinder flat head block and heaters under the seats. It sat in our outback for 20 years waiting to be rescued. -BJ

On Saturday evening, in Stovin's Lounge...

O n Saturday evening, in Stovin's Lounge, at the Bessborough Hotel, in Saskatoon:

• The man sitting beside me at the bar reaches across to the TV to turn up the sound for *Hockey Night in Canada*, changing from mute to barely audible. One of the servers comes over to him. He is on a high stool on the outside; she is on the inside. She bends close to him, subtle and quiet-voiced, and says, "The sound has to be kept off." I'm next to them, and I can barely hear what she is saying. The bar is relatively quiet; it's early. I don't take my eyes off the screen. "Not for Don Cherry, it doesn't," he says. "Cherry is an icon; we *have* to hear him." The server shrugs, laughs and walks away, leaving the sound at its forbidden audible level. On the TV, Grapes is wearing a kaleidoscopic, long, sparkly, cherry-red, fitted blazer. The world laughs and listens, all in one coordinated, rebellious, flowing motion.

• The bartender is the mother of three—ages 14, 12 and 9—and the man on the stool beside me has a 5-year-old son, adopted and blind.

I wonder if they knew he was blind when they adopted, but I don't ask. He reads my mind with ease and volunteers that they did not know and it is fine, your child is your child. I have daughters, age 25, I tell them. "Oh, they're twin," I say on seeing the puzzled looks regarding the same age. We compare parental notes, all the while serving drinks, eating supper, writing, answering cell phones, and watching the Leafs whip Ottawa.

• When Cherry finishes dispensing wisdom, the man beside me turns off the sound. He has just driven through a blizzard, on a business trip. "Me, too," I say and tell of yesterday having driven 900 kilometres in the same snow-burst in order to stay overnight at St. Peter's Benedictine monastery, in Muenster, northeast of Saskatoon. He doesn't ask why, and I don't volunteer. We drink to our bravery, complete with the obligatory self-mockery. He's into red wine, and I'm sipping Jameson's Irish Whiskey. He travels often and misses his family. Me, too. We toast the ones we love, again, and hope they appreciate us and the hardships we endure. The bartender smiles with us.

• This bartender is skilled. She works quickly and with accuracy, friendliness, and (bonus) humour. I know this game, and it is a pleasure doing business with her. There are several waiters to supply from the connected Japanese restaurant as well as her own bar and floor servers. It becomes a busy Saturday night, and her radar never stops. She conducts the ongoing scans without noise or fuss. She has just completed her Masters in Philosophy and is debating the worth of the ongoing PhD route, especially with three kids and being a single parent. She thinks she'll wait a couple of years, for the teenage storms and her debts to blow through, and then go to work on the doctorate, bartending in the evening. I don't ask if eventually she will quit tending bar. Why would I? More to the point, why would she?

• We three are versatile, and we complement each other. We have created a line—left winger, center and right winger—with our different attitudes, skills and roles becoming evident as we make the passes and take and deflect the shots. For this one night, we are playing for the same team, and our different ages, histories and appearances aren't important. We're pleased to be in this game together, for a few shifts anyway.

• The Leafs win 5—1, and I finish my meal; it's almost time to go. I wind up with a sorbet and a cognac, deep into recovery from the self-denial rigours of the monastery. The bartender and the bar companion and I smile and meet eyes and wish each other good trips, good times. Our line probably won't get to play together again, and we know it; such is the expected lot of all-star teammates. We did what we came to do, what we are paid to do, and the fans got their money's worth.

In October I was visiting a friend...

*I*n October I was visiting a friend in the Maritimes, a best kind of friend, but I was having trouble being open to connection, the sharing of place and talk, to being a friend of good heart. This happens, and usually I can do something about it, once I recognize the signs and (this is the difficult part) if I want to.

I *did* want to, so stayed up late to have a talk with myself, to get a grip. It was well after midnight, and I was still chasing mental and emotional weaves and dodges, slowly untying myself from my own knots, when I decided to turn on the radio, CBC 2, which I continue to call "CBC FM." Ross Porter was on, much later in the Maritimes I realized, and he used most of his show to play Marc Jordan's then-new CD, *This Is How Men Cry*, a serious and sensitive exploration of our need to get along with each other, carefully. I listened and felt that I heard the songs, the message, and went to bed feeling easier with myself, the solitary self and the caring self, both. I also felt easier with my friend.

Later on, in the weeks and eventually months that followed, I occasionally visited sound stores in Winnipeg, Kenora, Calgary, and Toronto, looking for the CD but not finding it. Just before Christmas I was in a large store in Winnipeg, early in the morning, again looking and again not finding. The store was almost empty. I spoke across a rack and an aisle to an employee, asking if she knew ". . . where Marc Jordan's new CD, *How Men Cry*, is?" She didn't and motioned me to follow her to the computer so we could search, modern style. As she was tapping in the information, I became aware of a man standing behind me. He said, "Excuse me; where did you hear of that Marc Jordan CD?"

"On Ross Porter's CBC night show. He played it a couple of months ago, and it's great. His show is called…I forget…"

"Late Night With…," he started to say, and by now he was grinning.

"*You're* Ross Porter! Right? I've never seen you, but I don't know how I missed that voice at first."

We shook hands after I told him how much I enjoyed his work, leaving out the fact that he should be charging therapeutic fees, not wanting to spook him, not with that voice. Some things you do *not* tamper with.

The woman using the computer found the CD for me, and I bought three. There are messages that must be shared.

A friend writes, from Prince Edward Island...

A friend writes from Prince Edward Island:

"I'm just back from a walk in the road to the dead-end where there are several houses tucked in the woods, and a couple of notices warning of children playing. Having been well announced by some barking dogs, I was soon joined by three kids—two on bikes and one on foot with two dogs—so I told them I was 'new to the road' and living in the blue house.

'Oh, we were wondering who moved in there,' and

'Do you have any pets? Because Daniel has eleven kittens.'

Well, I told Thomas, the walker and brother of Robyn on her bike, that I was looking for places to walk and did he know of any. So, after a short conference they decided I should be taken to the old dam, whereupon Daniel, the youngest, balanced himself barefoot on his bike, turned his big brown eyes to me and stated, 'It'th a peathful plathe.' I tell you, he stole my heart.

And, indeed, it is. They also told me about another potential walk and where to catch frogs and a good place to skate in winter and where I could get my lawn-mower fixed and where the osprey nest is. So, I'm making friends, on the road."

Montreal's souterrain, the subway Metro...

Montreal's souterrain, the subway Metro, runs relatively quietly on rubber tires along routes named for the end-point terminals—Henri-Bourassa, Côte-Vertu, Angrignon, Saint-Michel, Longueuil, Snowdon, and Honoré-Beaugrand. For several decades I have visited Montreal, alone and with friends, to watch the Montreal Expos Baseball Club play. I usually boarded the Metro at Atwater, Peel or McGill stations, riding to the Olympic Stadium stop at Pie-IX.

From this 'pee-neuf' exit, or 'pie-9' for the stubbornly anglo, it was a crowded but brief and gently uphill indoor walk to the Big-O's inner gates, with a couple of pauses en route to support the city's scalper, busker and panhandler economies. Since the 1970s, I've made this trip about fifty times. Today, I'm sorry to be making it for the last time.

Benita and I have heard CBC radio's Sports Report commenting that there will be a closing-out sale of all remaining Expos' items at the Olympic Stadium Boutique, as the team has been moved to a new city and country and taken on a new name. We ride the subway to Pie-IX. When we get off, there is a square ceramic tile high on the Metro wall, with a white background fronted by an Expos insignia and a bonus arrow pointing toward the Stadium. Someone has tried to erase or deface the symbols but have only partially succeeded, as the result is smudged and blurry but still legible. We walk with ten or twelve widely spaced others up the ramp to the closing-out. The route is familiar despite several years of my neglect, me and a few million others. The Expos are finished, but it appears that some of us are not, at least a few of us are not.

Ben and I and about ten people cruise the mostly empty aisles of the small store, which is an indoor, windowed island immediately opposite the entry gates to the O. There's very little talking. We buy Expos-labelled t-shirts and pencils, a 2004 Season Guide, which is the last one and contains snippets of the more valued past, a small Expos change purse, and a few no-message team cards in red envelopes. We try on caps, but they don't fit, not even those of the right size. A plastic batting helmet is lifted, held and replaced on the shelf.

As we walk away, even more slowly, we see an old man sitting on the tiled floor with his back against the tunnel wall, near the entry to the Metro station. Over his head and along the tunnel-ramp walls are the still-lit but now empty large, rectangular photo-display boxes, which used to have player images. These were action photos of Tim Wallach, Andre Dawson, Gary Carter, Tim Raines, Ellis Valentine, Warren Cromarte, Larry Walker, Dennis Martinez, Jeff Reardon, Steve Rogers, Andreas Galarraga, Jose Vidro, and Vladimir Guerrero. At various times they were there.

The old man is skinny and bearded, and his clothes are ripped and dirty. We're about twenty metres apart, close enough to nod, smile and gesture friendly low-key waves. We continue walking, and he continues sitting. I hope he will ask for money. He doesn't.

In the Sioux Lookout airport...

I n the Sioux Lookout airport on a foggy November morning, the
tapestry is unfolding itself:

• Many flights are on hold because of freezing rain north of us.
While we wait, there is much wandering around the terminal, random
movement intended to combat boredom. The maneuver doesn't seem
to be effective, at a glance, but many of us persist;

• A long-haired woman working behind an airline counter is a
magnet for eyes, male and female, young and old; it doesn't matter; she
is an all-purpose magnet. She is wearing beige pants and a black short-
sleeved shirt, and most importantly she is wearing an attitude of being
calmly busy in the midst of chaos, seemingly oblivious to the attention
she is receiving;

• One or two people seem to be watching the watchers. It might
be more than one or two, as some others are either profoundly subtle
as they observe things, or they are in a pre-coma state;

• The Anishnabe women over age 60 are all wearing bright head-
scarves, and most have on dresses or skirts with floral prints. None

of the younger Anishnabe women are wearing scarves or dresses, and black is the colour of their day, of their generation;

• Many of the fifty or more waiting people do not appear to be bearing the boredom with graceful ease, not at all. These are an impatient, dejected, and restless group of wristwatch gazers and payphone addicts, not skilled at waiting. Some others, however, have a measured and non-intrusive way of walking and sitting and speaking. Perhaps there is a statement being made, based on thousands of years of knowledge, regarding the necessity of a reserved respect for individual space and shared time;

• I attempt to observe my own generalizations, gaffes, and internal frozen precipitations but postpone the effort until the rain eases;

• The announcements from the airlines, which may be vital to our day, are impossible to understand: *"ATTENTION, PUL-EEEZE! MXQRST OD OTTINSB SANDY LAKE AND QRNISS AB VX OTN!"* No one moves in either definitive direction, not toward the back-to-town door and not toward the to-the-airplane door, so the message *must* indicate a form of cohesiveness and possibly even potential movement. We wait in hope.

The eyes of the beholders all record the day in our own ways, over and over. The tapestry folds and unfolds. Freezing rain is a blessing.

Acknowledgements

Benita Cohen offers companionship, friendship and generosity; accepted with gratitude.

* * * * *

I have admired Bob Jeffery's work and life for years and appreciate having the opportunity to link images.

* * * * *

Karen Sinclair has again provided fine organizational and editorial input—thank you, KS.

* * * * *

Many of these pieces were first published in the *Kenora Enterprise*, and I appreciate that paper's episodic willingness to use images without context, an inclination that involves small-town risk.

-PS

Thanks to my mother, father and Fr. Hurkes for teaching me how to look, to see and to capture images. Tammy, thanks for sharing.

-BJ

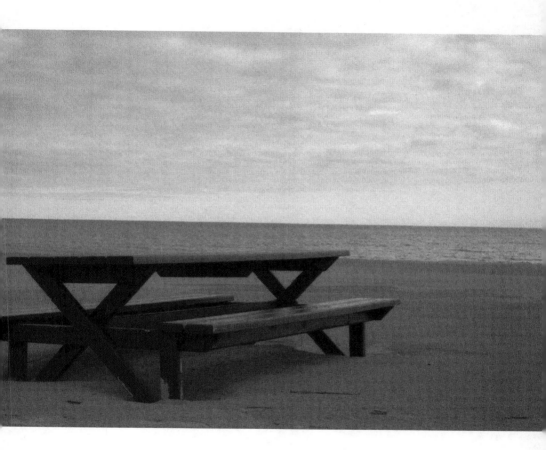

*In time the beach would consume this table; in the meantime people sit
and ponder as they gaze out at the water. -BJ*

Edwards Brothers Malloy
Oxnard, CA USA
February 20, 2013